OSTEOPOROSIS

Also in this series:

Bladder Problems
   Rosy Reynolds
Smear Tests
   Dr Jane Chomet and Julian Chomet
Trush
   Jane Butterworth
Pelvic Inflammatory Disease and Chlamydia
   Patsy Westcott
Anaemia
   Jill Davies
Breast Awareness
   Cath Cirket
Cystitis
   Dr Caroline Shreeve
Endometriosis
   Dr Lyle Brietkopf and Mavion Gordon Bakoulis
Fibroids
   Felicity Smart and Professor Stuart Campbell
Hormone Replacement Therapy
   Patsy Westcott

OSTEOPOROSIS

The brittle bones epidemic and how you can avoid it

Kathleen Mayes

Thorsons

An Imprint of HarperCollins*Publishers*

Thorsons
An Imprint of HarperCollins*Publishers*
77–85 Fulham Palace Road
Hammersmith, London W6 8JB

First published by Thorsons 1987
This revised new format edition published 1991
3 5 7 9 10 8 6 4

A catalogue record for this book
is available from the British Library

ISBN 0 7225 2509 5

Printed in Great Britain by
HarperCollins Manufacturing, Glasgow

Contents

List of Illustrations

List of Tables

ACKNOWLEDGEMENTS

This book would not have been possible without the valuable help and provision of reference material from many people and organizations. I am especially appreciative of the manuscript reviews done by:

Francis S. Johnson, D.D.S., Santa Barbara, California.

Robert Marcus, M.D., Stanford University School of Medicine, California.

Frederick Singer, M.D., Orthopedic Hospital, Los Angeles, California.

I also want to give my grateful thanks to:

Dorothy J. Bates, R.D., The American Dietetic Association, Chicago, Illinois.

Roberta DeVito, American Brittle Bone Society, West Chester, Pennsylvania.

Judi Greening, Frieda's Finest/Produce Specialities Inc., Los Angeles, California.

Ann Z. Grinham, Marion Laboratories Inc., Kansas City, Missouri.

M. Christine Hinsman, Lederle Laboratories, Wayne, New Jersey.

Norma J. Killila, Michigan Bean Commission, Lansing, Michigan.

Florence Kirk, R.D., California Milk Advisory Board, Modesto, California.

Alan E. Kligerman, LactAid, Inc., Pleasantville, New Jersey.

Beverly McKee, Dairy Council of California, Sacramento, California.

Paula M. Murphy, LICSW, Human Nutrition Research Center on Aging, Tufts University, Boston, Massachusetts.

Robert R. Recker, M.D., Department of Medicine, Creighton University, Omaha, Nebraska.
James L. Warren, Maine Sardine Council, Brewer, Maine.

And thanks also to:

Alaska Seafood Marketing Institute, Juneau, Alaska.
American Society for Bone and Mineral Research
California Dry Bean Advisory Board, Dinuba, California.
National Council on the Aging, Inc., Washington DC.
National Dairy Council, Division of Nutrition Education, Rosemont, Illinois.
National Digestive Diseases Education and Information Clearinghouse
National Institutes of Health, Bethesda, Maryland.
National Soft Drink Association, Washington, DC.
Washington State Dairy Council, Seattle, Washington.

AUTHOR'S NOTE

The use of brand names in this guide is for identification only and does not imply endorsement or otherwise by the author.

The calcium values in this guide have generally been obtained from McCance and Widdowson's *The Composition of Foods* by A.A. Paul and D.A.T. Southgate (H.M.S.O., 1978) and *Immigrant Foods*, the Second Supplement to 'The Composition of Foods' by S.P. Tan, *et al.* (H.M.S.O., 1985). Processing practices and formulas may vary from time to time, but the nutrient values are those currently available.

The author of this book wishes to emphasize that the contents are intended to inform readers, but are not intended to provide medical advice for individual ailments. Such advice should be sought from physicians. Before beginning any diet supplementation, it is recommended that you should consult with your doctor.

From 1959 to 1977 the numbers of hospital admissions for fracture of the neck of the femur increased by a factor of 2.7. Detailed analysis of data from the Hospital In-Patient Enquiry for 1968–77 showed that the increase applied to both sexes and at all ages over 45. . . The estimated number of admissions for men of all age groups increased by 55 per cent over the 10 years and for women this increase was 65 per cent. . .

Fracture of the neck of the femur has long been known as characteristic of aging; Sir Astley Cooper noted over 150 years ago the thinning of bones that accompanied aging. . .

Accelerated bone loss may have a hormonal or nutritional origin. . . There remains, however, the possibility that diminished activity in our society contributes to accelerated bone loss. Reasons for an increased frequency of falls give rise to even greater speculation. . . Alcohol consumption rises steadily, as does the use of drugs, particularly psychotropic drugs. . . Whatever the reason, the increase in need for hospital care to treat fracture of the neck of the femur has a major impact. . . The *additional* 16,000 admissions a year used about 600,000 bed-days at a cost of £40 million yearly. . .

A. Fenton Lewis, M.B., Ph.D., Senior Medical Officer, Department of Health and Social Security
(*British Medical Journal*, Vol. 283, 7 November 1981)

INTRODUCTION

Scene: Any busy high street.
A frail, bent old woman totters along slowly with a cane.
Is she your mother? Your older sister?
Or is it **you** in ten – twenty – thirty years?

Genetically, our bodies have changed little in 40,000 years, and maybe women's bodies were not meant to endure beyond their reproductive period. With increasing longevity, the problem of brittle fracturing bones is quickly approaching a crisis.

In England and Wales in 1981 there were more than 2400 people over the age of 100. By the year 2010 the postwar 'baby boomers' will give the population a sudden overlay of grey, a society of the elderly.

According the the Office of Population Censuses and Surveys, more than 9 million of the UK population are over the age of sixty-five, and of that number nearly 5½ million are women.

Maintaining health and vigour in later years may depend on where you live: certain parts of the world — the Caucasus region in the Soviet Republic of Georgia, Kashmir, and Vilacabamba high in the Andes of Ecuador — all claim many inhabitants of well over 100.

When humans first evolved, bodies were designed to last between twenty and thirty years. From around 3000 BC to AD 1900, there was a gain of about twenty-nine years in the average life span. The biological limit is somewhere between 110 and 120 years. Can we alter the fundamental ageing programme in our genes, through genetic manipulation? It may sound like science fiction, but it certainly is possible. There is still much more to know about the genes that regulate longevity.

Originally 'hunter-gatherers', human tribes roamed the forests and plains for fruits, fibrous plant materials, roots, nuts, berries –

and only small amounts of lean meat were consumed when the hunt was successful. Humans naturally exercised muscles to find nutrients in order to survive. Designed for the tropics, skin naturally absorbed the sun's rays in *clear* air.

Our lifestyle and nutrition have changed considerably – today most people inhabit cities, with varying degrees of pollution; many have sedentary occupations, and food is as close as the neighbourhood shops, reached by car or bus.

Modern medicine and science have made vast strides in combatting many infectious diseases, and the leading causes of illness and death now are chronic degenerative problems such as heart disease, cancer and osteoporosis. Many health problems can be prevented or alleviated by improved nutrition or a change in lifestyle.

For the past fifty years, the medical profession has officially regarded nutrition as unimportant. But the medical journal *The Lancet*, now reflects a reversal of this view in more recent articles, veering towards the opinion that nutrition should be a major concern for all of us. The Royal College of Physicians recommends that all adults should remain physically active throughout life – taking more exercise, eating more fibre and less fat and sugar.

According to Dr Robert Butler, former head of the US National Institute on Aging, and now Brookdale Professor of Geriatrics and Adult Development at Mount Sinai Medical Center, New York City: 'Physical fitness can't be stressed enough. You need a nutritive diet, and enough exercise to maintain good heart function and increase bone strength.'

A problem of particular importance to every woman is osteoporosis. It is not new: archaeologists excavating in Northern Chile found well-preserved mummies of the Chinchorro culture of 7000 years ago. Among the Chinchorro, 31 per cent of the population had osteoporosis, all sufferers being women and two-thirds of them were under forty.

Osteoporosis is now so common, reaching the proportions of an epidemic, that all women should want to adopt a lifetime of good nutrition and a lifestyle that will protect their bones. The affliction ranks close behind arthritis as a major chronic disease of older people, especially women, and yet to a large extent it could be prevented. Although there is much that scientists do not yet understand about this disorder, evidence suggests that simple changes in lifestyle may prevent, or at least slow down, its development. In many cases, it is needless and preventable!

The key to fighting osteoporosis is understanding what it is, knowing while you are still young if you may be at risk, and what you can do to lessen its effects.

The National Osteoporosis Society estimates that up to 10 per cent of women can expect a broken hip. There are up to 50,000 hip fractures (fractures of the neck of the femur) each year in Britain, especially among women past the menopause, with osteoporosis often the underlying cause. The additional cost of medical care in the United Kingdom (including private and National Health Service treatment) for patients with hip fractures is about £500 million each year.

Recent studies indicate the highest incidence of these fractures to be in Britain, New Zealand and Sweden. Many suffer from weakened vertebrae and may have chronic spinal problems. It is estimated that one-sixth of these victims die from ensuing complications of their fractures, and countless more are disabled permanently.

So the good news is that people in Western countries are living longer; the bad news is that osteoporosis is becoming a potential problem for greater numbers of women. The question facing each of us is how much we want to take charge to get the utmost out of our lives.

Chapter 1

WHAT IS OSTEOPOROSIS?

Os'-te-o-po-ro'-sis literally means porous bones, a reduction in the density along with increasing brittleness, associated with the decrease in calcium. Osteoporosis can affect the *strength* and the *amount* of bone tissue. The condition occurs as a normal part of ageing, but other factors can produce a crisis condition. As bones become thinner, they become more fragile and porous and are therefore more susceptible to fracturing. Bones can be so weak they can't stand up to everyday activity: a fall, a blow, or lifting action, that would not bruise or strain the average person, can easily break a bone in someone with severe osteoporosis. A simple action like making a bed, lifting a casserole out of the oven, or even an affectionate hug, can cause spinal fracture in a person with severe osteoporosis.

Research data collected by the US National Institute on Aging shows that women are more likely than men to suffer osteoporosis: 1 in 4 postmenopausal white women is affected by this bone-thinning, and 1 in 8 men over sixty. According to government statistics, about 25 per cent of all white women in America have had one fracture or more by the age of sixty-five, due largely to osteoporosis.

There are several types of osteoporosis:

- *Primary* (or *postmenopausal*) is an age-related disorder. It occurs mainly in older women, and can be due to many different underlying causes, chiefly heredity, poor nutrition, deficiency of hormones and lack of exercise.
- *Genetic* osteoporoses are linked with abnormalities of chromosomes controlling bone metabolism.
- *Immobilization* or *disuse* osteoporosis, which can be *localized*

when, for instance, a leg is paralyzed or put in a plaster cast, or *generalized* if you have prolonged bed-rest, paralysis, confinement to a wheelchair, or periods of weightlessness (as with astronauts).

● *Secondary* osteoporosis, suffered by men, women and children, generally caused by certain diseases or drugs.

Although osteoporosis can affect any of your bones, the disorder will usually first show up in the bones of your forearm and your spine. It can mean a loss in height of up to 1½ inches (3.75 cm) every ten years; severe cases can see a loss of up to 2 inches (5 cm) in a few weeks. Collapsed vertebrae can cause severe back pain, and with weakened jawbones and ligaments, teeth can be lost or loosened. Even with a loss of one-third of bone mass, porosity is not likely to show up on X-rays, so fractures in hips and wrists are often the first warning that bones are 'thinning'. The majority of fractures in the elderly occur in vertebrae, wrist, hip, shoulder and knee joints.

Spinal fractures

These mostly happen when a woman is between fifty and seventy, averaging about sixty years of age. Normal adult vertebrae are roughly rectangular, separated by intervertebral discs. The vertebrae of the spine are usually the first bones to show signs of osteoporosis, as they become porous and weakened and then deformed, with varying degrees of compression and wedging (see Figure 1). With the weight of your body to support, the bones of the spine can callapse, causing 'crush fractures', and when several vertebrae collapse, eventually the rib cage tilts down to rest on your hipbones. In this way, the upper spine curves outward (kyphosis), the lower spine inward (lordosis), producing the hunchback deformity known as 'dowager's hump'. When the ribs tilt down, they force the internal organs outward, causing severe pain in many cases, and the loss of several inches in height, in the upper part of the body (since the length of the arm- and leg-bones does not change).

Wrist fractures

These often occur when a woman over fifty falls and puts out her

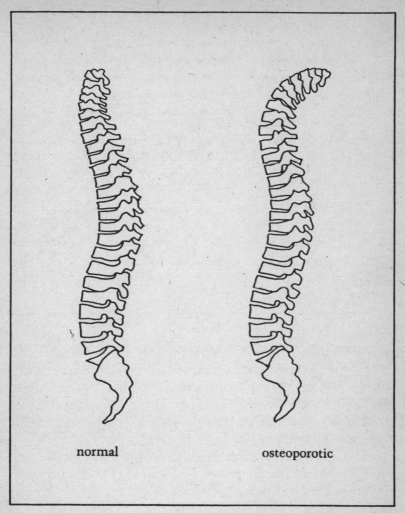

normal osteoporotic

Figure 1

arm to save herself. One type is called a 'Colles Fracture', associated with displacement of the ends of fractured forearm bones, usually the radii (see Figure 2). These fractures may act as a warning that bones are weakened, and a more serious hip fracture may ensue.

Hip fractures

Hip fractures generally affect older people, and are more frequent

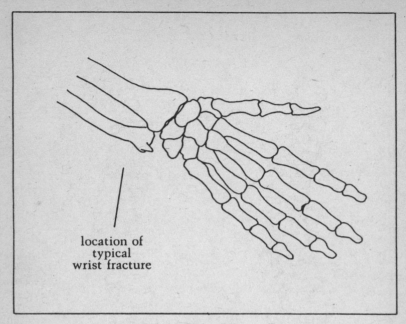

location of
typical
wrist fracture

Figure 2

in women than in men. The hip is the only true ball-and-socket joint in the body, and the largest joint except for the knee. When porous and brittle, the thigh bones are most vulnerable to fracturing, especially in the top at the hip socket where this part of the femur (the 'neck') is the narrowest and yet has to carry the full load of the upper body (see Figure 3).

Although fractures of the vertebrae can happen spontaneously, hip fractures are usually caused by an accident such as tripping over a small rug or slipping in the bath. Occasionally a hip fracture happens for no apparent reason, which triggers the thought – was the fall caused by a broken hip, or did the hip fracture because of the fall? A woman who has suffered a fractured hip on one side is twenty times more likely to have a subsequent fracture on the other.

Disabilities from such fractures are often the beginning of serious physical decline for the elderly: after leaving hospital, many osteoporotic patients are so afraid of falling that they lead very sedentary lives, depressed and full of despair at the disruption of their lives, remaining in nursing homes until death. Statistics

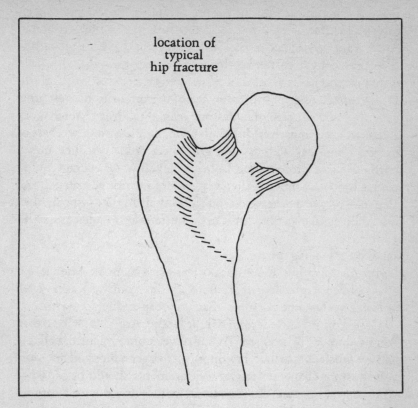

location of
typical
hip fracture

Figure 3

can be frightening: 15 per cent of women die shortly after a hip fracture; almost 30 per cent die within a year; less than 50 per cent are able to return to normal life. A wrist fracture can be disabling for two months, but long-term disability is not uncommon. A hip fracture is one of the leading causes of accidental death among elderly white women, reducing life expectancy by 12 per cent. The cause of death is not the fracture itself, but the result of ailments associated with prolonged nursing home or hospital stays — pneumonia, blood clots, or a fat embolism.

Do men suffer osteoporosis?

Although the condition in men has not been studied to the same extent as in women, they can and do suffer from it, though usually at a much later age with the normal decline of their overall bone mass. Among those who live to the age of ninety, 17 per cent of men will suffer a hip fracture. Look around any nursing home. Apart from age-related osteoporosis, they may have the secondary type caused by a particular drug or disease. Men can also have disuse osteoporosis as a result of prolonged bed-rest or paralysis. But generally osteoporotic men are in the minority because men have about 30 per cent greater bone mass at maturity, weigh more and have larger muscles. Unlike women, they have a slower rate of natural bone loss with ageing, without a sudden decline in sex hormones that protect their bones. They also, on average, don't live as long as women. However, where nutrition, exercise and alcoholism have a bearing on the risks involved for a woman, they would be similar factors for a man, but maybe to a lesser extent.

Are you losing bone?

Unfortunately, because osteoporosis is a silent disease, it has always been a problem that there are few outward signs until bones have become so weak that they can suddenly fracture.

Have you measured your height lately? Are you shorter than you used to be, or stooped? As spinal vertebrae fracture, collapse and are crushed together, height is lost between hips and neck and your posture changes. Height measurements should be a part of your routine medical examinations, with every doctor's surgery having a scale on the wall for measurements to be made regularly. Do you know how tall you were at skeletal maturity, about the age of twenty-five? You can roughly calculate your early adult height by measuring your armspan, since that width is usually (but not always) nearly equal to your earlier height at adulthood. Deduct this armspan measurement from your present head-to-heel height for a rough estimate of height loss.

Do you have transparent skin? On the back of your hand, if the skin is loose and lacking pigment so you can see the edges of small as well as large veins, this transparency indicates collagen deficiency in the outer layers of your skin. As one of the components of bone is collagen, it has been concluded that skin thickness has a correlation with bone thickness. However, this is also an indication of rheumatoid arthritis. Skin thickness can be measured with calipers in your doctor's surgery.

Do you have gum disease? Gum disease *can* be a sign of poor dental hygiene – but sometimes it is a warning of osteoporosis. Many adults, especially middle-aged women, lose their teeth with pyorrhoea. Periodontal disease or pyorrhoea affects the tissues supporting your teeth – the gums, ligaments attaching teeth to your jaw and sometimes the alveolar bone. Where there is loss of bone in the jaw, gums can recede, teeth are not securely held in their proper place and change position, inviting bacteria to the exposed areas between gums and teeth. If too much alveolar ridge is lost, even dentures cannot be properly seated. Ask your dentist about X-rays of your jaw as they can be a useful indication of the bone density elsewhere in your body.

If you think your bones may be at risk, other tests can be done to evaluate bone mass, depending to some extent on the equipment available in your neighbourhood, and how your physician prefers to approach the problem. Sometimes doctors will take blood and urine samples for analyses of calcium in the blood and calcium excreted in urine and thus lost from your body. These tests do not provide a diagnosis of primary osteoporosis with any degree of certainty, because of variations resulting from food intake, metabolism, heavy use of laxatives, and the possibility of other bone disease.

Although spinal, hip and jawbone X-rays are frequently used, they are perhaps not sufficiently sensitive to discern early bone loss, the problem being that in standard X-ray imaging the hard dense outer layer of bone tissue (cortical bone) can hide the inner honeycomb-type bone (trabecular bone). With osteoporosis, cortical bone gets thinner, and trabecular bone more porous, but unless 30 per cent of bone mass is lost, radiologists might have difficulty in detecting osteoporosis. In some cases, X-rays may reveal that one or more vertebrae have already fractured, even though you have not been conscious of any back pain. Many patients with osteoporosis do have pain, however: either a chronic ache along the spine or pain from spasm in the back muscles. This occurs when the muscles of the back must take an increased share of the load of supporting the upper half of the body, after the spine has partially collapsed. Then the muscles will 'complain' periodically.

If you live in a large city or near a big hospital, the preferred method of evaluation is a CAT scan. Computerized Axial Tomography is a way of seeing bones with multiple X-ray exposures combined by computer into one picture. By modifying a CAT scanner, which produces a cross-sectional image of your body, or part of your body, doctors can get a reading on the amount of bone density. A modified scanner, differentiating and separating images of trabecular (where bone loss is more severe) and cortical bone, can tell the amount of bone mineral present, whether there is some degree of osteoporosis, and monitor it so there are no further complications.

In certain clinics, it may be possible to have tests using other types of X-ray equipment: radiogrammetry, radiographic photo-densitometry or photon absorptiometry, to measure bones in fingers or forearms, since if you do have osteoporosis it will be occurring in many places simultaneously.

Single photon absorptiometry measures the density of forearm bones or the heel. The bone is penetrated by a narrow beam of photons from a radioactive source. Radiation exposure is quite low, under 10mrem. This test is useful if you are over 75, and if you have had large changes in bone density due to medical treatments.

Dual photon absorptiometry is similar, except that the radioactive source produces two beams, for a more precise measurement. It can be used to measure the hip, the spine and other skeletal sites. Radiation exposure is about 30mrem. This test is appropriate if you are middle-aged, because it measures the hip and spine. However, it is less useful than a CAT scan if you are over 75 or have calcium deposits or bone degeneration around the spine.

Dual energy radiography is still being developed, but promises greater precision and lower radiation. Total body neutron activation analysis, performed in a very few research laboratories, is a method for measuring the total calcium in your body, and your skeleton in particular.

If your doctor considers further examination necessary, he will investigate what is available in your area, what diagnostic equipment is in nearby clinics, hospitals and research centres, and the costs involved if you have private treatment. Usually at least two separate tests are necessary, to discover the rate at which your body is being depleted of calcium and your rate of bone loss.

Chapter 2

ABOUT YOUR BONE STRUCTURE

An essential part of a human being is the skeleton. The word 'skeleton' comes from the Greek meaning 'dried up', because by itself, the skeleton looks like a completely dried up human, or a shrivelled mummy without skin (or so the Greeks thought). The skeleton is about 18 per cent of your weight – about 25 pounds (11 kg), made up of 206 separate bones to support and protect your body:

long, like the thigh bones, for example,
short, like the wrist bones,
flat, like your ribs, and
irregular, like your vertebrae.

Almost every bone is designed to fit a particular need, with a notable exception being the coccyx, Man's vestigial tail.

The common name for the bones that run down your back is 'backbone', which may sound like a single bone, although twenty-six articulated bones are involved in an adult, held together and kept upright by muscles and ligaments. Another common name is 'spinal column' or spine, which again suggests a single bone. But if the spine were a single bone, your back would be completely stiff and unable to bend – like your thigh bone, which *is* one long piece. The spinal column is composed of many bones, separated by discs of fibre and cartilage that act as shock absorbers, enabling your trunk to turn to either side, bend backwards or forwards, or even in small circular movements. It doesn't bend at one point, like the elbow in your arm, but slightly at several points. Because the spinal column can bend in different directions, its formal name is vertebral column, from the Latin 'vertere', to turn. So each individual bone in the vertebral column is called a vertebra, which is how our division of the animal kingdom came to be called vertebrates.

At birth, there are two curves in the vertebral column as in typical land-vertebrates: a downward curve at the neck and an upward curve in the back. So babies crawl. But during the second year, a child rises on hind legs, finding it increasingly easy, comfortable and natural like that. The vertebral column gradually bends back in the hip region to form a new curve that is shaped towards the back. The human spine, though still straight when seen from behind, now has a kind of double-S shape when seen from the side. The curves of the spine make it easy to keep upright and give a springy balance. Other animals, such as bears and gorillas, do not have this spinal curve in the region of the hip, so they can't maintain an upright position for long.

Bone tissue consists of tiny particles of *calcium* and *phosphorus* in a network of *collagen* fibres. The calcium gives strength and hardness to bones, without which your bones would be like jelly. The collagen gives a certain amount of flexibility. Your bones also naturally contain fluoride, sodium, potassium, magnesium, citrate, plus other trace elements – all helping to hold the calcium and phosphorus building-blocks together.

The body of a 154 pound (70 kg) man contains about 2½ pounds (1.2kg) of calcium – between 1.5 and 2 per cent of his total body weight.

Bone tissue is a storehouse for your reserves of calcium, containing 99 per cent of the calcium in your body, to be added to or withdrawn from as needed to maintain a balance of calcium in the blood. The other 1 per cent of calcium is found in soft tissues and fluids throughout your body, with the level of calcium in the blood kept fairly constant, as required for muscle contraction, pulse rate and heart contractions, normal blood clotting and brain functioning. When blood levels of calcium become low, calcium is resorbed from the bones to help keep up blood calcium. When blood levels of calcium return to normal, bone resorption slows down.

Bones manufacture blood cells; they are tissues with blood vessels, nerve fibres and fluid-filled channels.

Like other body tissues, living bone is always being rebuilt, *bone remodelling* is constantly under way: new bone is formed on the outer surfaces while small quantities of old bone on the inner surfaces are lost through breakdown and resorbed by the body. A bone-making cell is called an *osteoblast* and in its mature form in the bone it is called an *osteocyte*, important in the nutrition and maintenance of normal bone. The bone-resorbing cell which is responsible for remodelling and reshaping bones during growth and repair is called an *osteoclast*. The delicate balance maintained between these processes is your *bone mass* – the total amount in your skeleton – a balance that is always changing according to your body needs, affected by heredity, diet, drugs, physical activity, hormones, stress, injury and disease.

Basically, there are two different types of bone tissue: *cortical* and *trabecular* (see Figure 4). Cortical bone is very solid and dense, and is mostly in the long hard bones of arms and legs. Trabecular bone looks rather like a honeycomb, though much more porous, and this type is mostly in the spinal vertebrae. Each bone has both types of material, with the solid cortical bone on the outside as a

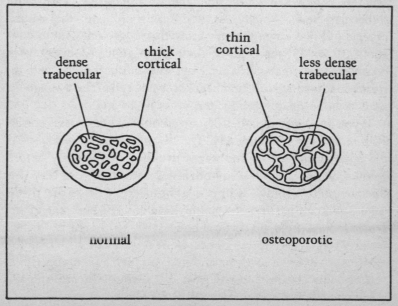

Figure 4

shell around the spongy trabecular kind in the interior. The proportions of cortical and trabecular bone vary, depending on which bone it is and which part of the bone. Normally, at the 'neck' of the femur it is about 50 per cent cortical, 50 per cent trabecular. The lower part of the radius is about 75 per cent cortical, 25 per cent trabecular. Vertebrae are about 10 per cent cortical, 90 per cent trabecular.

The spongy bone in the inside of long bones forms a system of great strength – sufficient to carry loads with an economy of material. If your bones were all completely solid, your skeleton would be impossibly heavy and yet not have much more structural strength than it actually does. But it is trabecular bone tissue which is most susceptible to changes that occur in bone remodelling.

Bone tissue is formed when the human embryo is only two months old, then built up through childhood and adolescence until you are about twenty-five to thirty years old. When you are young, the build-up of bone growth predominates over breakdown; your bones get larger and more dense up to maturity. In adulthood the two processes are in equilibrium. Peak bone mass for cortical bone is reached at about the age of thirty-five, earlier for trabecular bone. Finally, as you reach old age, the natural process of breakdown prevails more than regrowth. Adults have about 10 to 15 per cent of their bone replaced every year, according to estimates, in a cycle of three to four months, with the formation, maintenance and breakdown of cells. The average life span of bone tissue is about ten years in an adult.

If you live long enough, a certain amount of bone loss is normal – about 0.5 per cent annually. The decline of trabecular bone in the spine can start in the early twenties, particularly among women, with a slight loss in both sexes until the age of fifty. But the rate can be as much as 1 per cent or more a year, so that by the time a woman is fifty, she might have lost 30 per cent of her skeletal mass. Loss of cortical bone starts in the early thirties, mostly from arm- and leg-bones. Bone loss can be accelerated if muscles are inactive, as with paralyzed patients, by prolonged bed-rest or being confined to a wheelchair. Certain diseases can also accelerate decline in bone mass.

How do you make your bones?

Calcium is a vital part of bone formation and the replacement of bone cells, with a system of hormones making sure you always have sufficient calcium in your blood, storing reserves of calcium in your bones, or stimulating its excretion.

Bone growth is controlled by many different factors, depending on your age and sex, in a delicate system of signals between the pituitary gland and other glands in your endocrine system. Most important is the growth hormone from the pituitary gland, with the sex hormones (oestrogens and progesterone in girls, androgens in boys) and thyroid hormones, adrenal glands, parathyroid glands and vitamin D. During the acceleration of sex hormone production in adolescence, there is a surge of growth at both the inner and outer surfaces of bone tissue.

Growth hormone. Especially active in your early years, this hormone produced by the pituitary gland triggers tissue growth, including bone-forming cartilage. The effect of growth hormone is controlled by hormones in your liver, conveyed via the bloodstream to the growing areas of your skeleton. Research is continuing on the role of growth hormone in adults.

Thyroid hormones. These hormones are also important for determining the proper formation of your skeletal mass in early years, with a deficiency resulting in dwarfed development and an excess resulting in a stimulation of bone remodelling and hence bone loss.

Parathyroid hormone. Four parathyroid glands in your neck near the thyroid gland release parathyroid hormone into your bloodstream regulating calcium in your blood when it falls too low. A signal is given to your kidneys to return to the bloodstream the calcium that otherwise would be sent to the urine. This hormone can also convert vitamin D to an active form, so that your intestines can absorb more calcium from your food. Parathyroid can also stimulate the breakdown of bone to maintain calcium levels in your bloodstream.

Vitamin D. This is now considered a hormone rather than a vitamin. It comes mostly from the ultraviolet rays in sunshine (or from an ultraviolet lamp) on your skin, producing an inactive form of vitamin D. Small quantities are also in foods such as milk, eggs and fish. The vitamin is stored in fatty tissues in your liver, and sent to the kidneys where it is converted to an active form. Activated vitamin D increases the absorption of calcium from food in the intestines and the reabsorption of calcium through the kidneys. Similar to the parathyroid hormone, D maintains the calcium-phosphorus levels in the bloodstream. However, if D is present in excessively high levels, it can extract calcium from the bones, causing bone loss. Vitamin D is beneficial in the right amounts, but too much can have the reverse effect and you could lose bone unnecessarily.

Calcitonin. This is a hormone released mainly by the thyroid gland, to balance the harmful effects of parathyroid and activated vitamin D. Men have more calcitonin than women, which is perhaps why they are more protected from bone loss.

Oestrogen and Progesterone. The ovaries of a premenopausal woman produce oestrogen in the first part of the menstrual cycle and progesterone in the second half. Small quantities of oestrogen are also derived from the transformation of androgens (from ovaries and adrenals) to oestrogen in fat. Oestrogen seems to have a special influence on bone substance, slowing down the bone destruction process and improving the absorption of calcium from food by the intestines – although scientists are not sure of oestrogen's exact role.

Testosterone. This male sex hormone, produced by men in the testes, develops, protects and maintains the strength of bones in men in the same way that the female sex hormones, oestrogen and progesterone, do in women. However, men have a gradual decline in their production of testosterone and no menopause to bring about a rapid depletion.

Adrenal glands. A negative force on bone can occur when adrenal glands are overactive (or when drugs similar to the adrenal hormones, such as cortisone, have to be taken over an extended period of time). These glands near the kidneys are usually triggered by stress, both physical and emotional, and can accelerate the destructive effects of parathyroid hormone and excessive vitamin D.

So now look at a 'balance sheet' of some of the hormones involved in bone formation:

On the positive side	On the negative side
Growth hormone from the pituitary.	Deficiency of the growth hormone.
Calcitonin from the thyroid.	Excess activity in the thyroid.
Vitamin D from liver and kidneys.	Excess parathyroid.
Oestrogen and progesterone from ovaries (in women).	Excess activity in the adrenals.
Testosterone from testes (in men).	Insufficient oestrogen and progesterone.

At *menopause*, a different 'balance sheet' occurs. Menopause (or climacteric or 'change of life') is part of the natural process of ageing in women. At the beginning of the twentieth century, menopause in Western Europe occurred at about an average age of forty-four, but now the average age is fifty. It may be quite sudden or a gradual stage, with the decline of activity in the ovaries when they produce insufficient oestrogen and menstruation stops. In the years preceding natural menopause, the ovaries stop making progesterone (the hormone produced in the second half of the menstrual cycle) before they reduce their production of oestrogens.

If a younger woman has had the surgical removal of the uterus *and ovaries*, she undergoes a surgical menopause with an abrupt cessation of bone-protecting hormones.

While ovaries are still making oestrogens, the oestrogen continues to block the action of the parathyroid, and a woman who has undergone natural menopause will still produce the small amounts derived from androgens. But with lower oestrogen levels, bone can be vulnerable with reduced protection.

Bone loss can be accelerated for the first five or six years after menopause, whether natural or surgical, the breakdown of bone tissue being the reverse of the growth spurt during teenage years, with the rate finally slowing down at around the age of sixty-five. By this time a woman may have lost close to a half of her skeletal mass. Postmenopausal women also have a slower and declining function in kidneys and liver, resulting in a reduced ability to utilize the stored vitamin D. Extra calcium is extracted from storage in the bones, and more calcium is excreted than is taken in.

Chapter 3

WILL YOU BE A VICTIM?
Some Risks You Cannot Change

With the frightening statistics now emerging, all women have to ask themselves if they could become victims of osteoporosis. What are *your* chances of having bone thinning and fracturing? With roughly 1 in 4 women being affected, we are on the verge of an epidemic. The disorder is far more common in women than in men for many reasons. For instance:

- Women have smaller bones, with less bone mass at maturity.
- They get less exercise, so their muscles are smaller.
- They are inclined to go on slimming diets that frequently are not nutritionally balanced.
- Extra demands are made on their total calcium level during pregnancy and breast-feeding – an especially critical situation when teenage girls become pregnant before their bones have reached their peak mass.
- Women are taking up smoking in ever-increasing numbers.
- Alcoholism among women is on the increase.
- Many women are heavy users of laxatives.
- Many women take diuretics to flush water from their systems.
- More women are in stressful occupations in difficult jobs or have conditions at home that cause strain.
- More women are using antacids to overcome stomach problems.
- Hysterectomy, with removal of ovaries, is a common type of operation for women.
- After menopause, women no longer have the oestrogen hormones that have been giving bone protection.

• Women live longer than men, with an extension of life
  expectancy twenty-five or thirty years after menopause.

How much are *you* at risk? With many factors involved, it is not
easy to predict who will suffer. Some factors you can change, and
others such as gender and genes you obviously cannot. While a
certain amount of bone loss is normal, some factors play their part
in maintaining your bone mass, other factors have a bearing on
how quickly you lose it, and it also depends on how long you live.
Let's first consider some of the risk factors you *cannot* change.

Skin colour
Skin pigmentation is related to risk: the fairer your complexion,
the greater your risk. Fewer black people than white suffer
osteoporosis, because they tend to have about 10 per cent greater
bone mass at skeletal maturity, and larger muscles that create
greater stress on their bones. Blacks may have higher levels of
calcitonin in their systems. And studies have shown that white
women tend to lose more calcium in their urine than black
women. But when a black woman has had an early surgical
menopause, she can be at the same risk as a white woman who has
had the same surgery. When dark-skinned people live in northern
latitudes with fewer hours of sunshine, or under smoggy or cloudy
skies, they too can be at risk.

Racial differences
As studies continue on osteoporosis, it appears that you are *more*
likely to develop it if you were born in, or if your ancestors came
from –
    The British Isles
    Northern Europe
    China and Japan
    Arctic Eskimos of Canada and Alaska
And you are *less* likely to develop osteoporosis if your lineage is
from –
    Africa
    Mediterranean countries
    Australian aboriginals
Jewish women are somewhere in between low-risk blacks and

high-risk whites. In general, small-boned Caucasian and Oriental women are most susceptible to osteoporosis.

Bone mass at maturity

If you are petite, and have the same rate of bone loss as a larger woman, you will be at risk sooner, simply because you had less bone when you reached the peak of maturity. If you are a small-boned woman, regardless of body weight, you could be in danger.

What is your family history of osteoporosis?

Did your grandmother, mother, aunt or older sister suffer from it? Did they become noticeably shorter or more stooped as they grew older? (Think not only of your mother's side of the family, as you have genes from your father also.) If so, your chances are high of developing it too, unless you take preventive steps to protect your bones. In some families there can be a definite inherited link concerning the amount of bone mass achieved at maturity, a reduced amount of oestrogen produced by ovaries, and the rate of bone loss in later years. Simply by living longer, you can expect more bone loss to occur.

Age when menopause occurs

Generally, the sooner you experience your menopause, the greater your chances of osteoporosis.

Most women in industrial societies today undergo menopause between the ages of forty-five and fifty-four, with fifty currently being the median age. With the expectation of life now stretching out to thirty years beyond menopause, women are unprotected by oestrogens for a longer time.

Is there any way to tell when menopause will occur? There is no accurate way to predict it. If you started menstruating at an early age, it does not follow that you will stop any sooner. But the age at which menopause occurs does tend to run in families, so ask your mother, aunts, or older sisters, when they experienced menopause. If most did so in their early forties, you can expect a similar pattern; on the other hand, if they were menstruating into their fifties, you will probably do the same.

Have your ovaries been removed?

In some surgical cases, it is essential to remove ovaries because they are either diseased or damaged, but unfortunately some physicians routinely recommend healthy ovaries be taken out at the time of hysterectomy if a woman is approaching natural menopause anyway. They reason that such surgery would prevent possible ovarian cancer at a later date – a cancer which is often fatal because it is difficult to diagnose early. But removal of ovaries before natural menopause involves abrupt loss of oestrogens and a 50 per cent risk of the rapid onset of osteoporosis if hormone replacement therapy is not prescribed.

Christopher E. Cann, Ph.D. of the University of California at San Francisco, recently conducted a three-year study of forty-seven women (white-, yellow-, and brown-skinned), aged between twenty-four and forty-eight who had undergone oophorectomies (removal of ovaries). His report revealed that they lost spinal mineral content at an alarming average rate of 9 per cent the first year after the operation. Two women had lost more than 20 per cent!

There are several kinds of hysterectomies and it is important to know the differences:

Partial hysterectomy means the removal of the uterus and cervix.

Subtotal hysterectomy is the removal of the uterus but not the cervix.

Total hysterectomy or *hysterectomy and bilateral salpingo oophorectomy* is the removal of uterus, tubes and ovaries.

Hysterectomy and unilateral salpingo oophorectomy is the removal of one tube and one ovary.

Radical hysterectomy is the removal of tubes, ovaries, uterus, cervix and pelvic lymph nodes.

When a woman undergoes a partial hysterectomy or has only one ovary removed, her levels of hormones are usually unchanged. But a total or radical hysterectomy involving the extraction of both ovaries can cause a sudden cessation of hormone production with consequent severe menopausal symptoms, especially if the operation is performed when the woman is young or several years before natural menopause would have occurred.

In 1981, 63,620 women in England and Wales underwent

hysterectomy, and over 650,000 women in the United States had the surgery in the same year. Various surveys in the US have revealed that between 20 to 40 per cent are performed unnecessarily or for doubtful reasons. In some cases, it is used as a method of birth control, or as a way to correct menstrual irregularity, but this is a major operation, and simpler alternatives are often available. It is important to get a second opinion if your physician suggests a hysterectomy, to ensure that the surgery is essential; and it is crucial to know if both ovaries will be removed, as this will effect a surgical menopause, change your hormone level, and may trigger a rapid loss of bone mass. If ovaries are healthy, there are compelling reasons for leaving them intact – know your condition as thoroughly as possible *before* the operation.

Other chronic diseases

When medication is prescribed by your physician for other diseases or conditions, these additional factors can contribute to bone loss. For instance:

- Certain drugs, such as cortisone for rheumatoid arthritis and asthma; heparin (an anticoagulant) for heart disease and high blood pressure; diuretics for oedema; some antacids for acute indigestion; anticonvulsants for epileptic seizures.
- Disorders such as hyperthyroidism and kidney disease.
- Destruction of bone cells by radiation treatment or chemotherapy.
- Inability to absorb calcium from the intestine (severe ulcers or through the removal of part of your stomach).
- Excessive excretion of calcium in the urine (idiopathic hypercalciuria).
- Scoliosis (spinal curvature).

Discuss drugs with your doctor to see if dosage could be reduced, or if alternative medicine is available that would be less conducive to bone loss. For instance, if you take heparin, ask your doctor if you could change to a warfarin-type anticoagulant. If you take steroids for arthritis, would one of the new nonsteroid drugs be as effective for you? At the same time, ask your physician about calcium supplementation or other bone-promoting therapy that would be appropriate for your condition.

Chapter 4

YOU CAN BE IN CONTROL!

In many cases, osteoporosis is *preventable*! After looking at some of the factors and conditions that are unavoidable, let's see where you can be more in control of the situation – where you can exercise options that will reduce your risk of bone loss, and banish the apathetic feeling that it is an inevitable part of ageing. Some factors have a greater bearing on demineralization than others, depending on your food habits and lifestyle.

Do you eat well?

Hippocrates once said: 'Thy food shall be thy cure', and perhaps he was on the right track. The quality of your life can depend on the quality of your food. Some foods, or lack of them, can cause diseases; others prevent them. A sensible diet may add years to your life. There's no doubt, diet has an influence. Food is not a preventive nor a cure for *all* human diseases, but more is being learned about the interaction of food on health, and how much is needed to give a full and happy life span. Sometimes the only difference between a healthy person and a sick person is the food eaten. When poorly nourished and abused, your body gets out of order, you can get sick, and might age and die needlessly prematurely. There's still much you can do for yourself with preventive health practices and better nutrition. It's a combination of the right living habits, the right food and ways of preparing food, knowing which foods to avoid and which supplements may be needed. For fitness and the longest life span, you need a lifetime concern for good nutrition. But it's never too late to start on a programme of self-improvement, with the key points being: moderation in quantity, attention to quality, and especially a *variety* of items from the four main food groups – milk and milk products; fruits and vegetables; breads and cereals; meat, fish, poultry, eggs or beans. As no individual item contains all the nutrients you need, an assortment of whole food makes for better health.

As a mother, you probably feel your family's needs come first, and urge your youngsters to drink their milk or fruit juice and eat their vegetables, but make sure you too have your proper share of these foods.

Frequently, young people as well as the elderly, have to work with a limited budget for food. You may be bored with food and its preparation, or be in a hurry, or have little appetite, especially if you are living on your own. You may have difficulty chewing because of poor teeth or ill-fitting dentures, or have problems of indigestion. Or it may not be easy for you to get to the shops if you live some distance away from them, so you may not have much fresh food and choices may be limited or unwise. As years go by, you are probably less active and need fewer calories, but every calorie has to provide good sound nutrition and really count. There's little room for the 'empty calories' in fats, sugars and alcohol. Each day can make different demands on your body and the nourishment it needs, with varying levels of activity, days of stress and days of relaxation.

For determining good bone health, it is crucial to consume sufficient *calcium*, largely found in dairy products, especially during adolescence and young adulthood, and to have the right ratio of calcium to other foodstuffs. In Yugoslavia, a study of women's bone mass was conducted in two villages in regions of the country with different eating habits, one group consuming twice as much calcium as the other. In the village where calcium consumption was high, the women's bones were definitely stronger at skeletal maturity, and fewer fractures were suffered by the elderly. It has been found that women with osteoporosis have generally had poor nutrition, with less calcium, or have had difficulty in absorbing it from their food. As we grow older, it can become more difficult to absorb calcium. Later on, you will read of the different foods that are calcium-rich and the role played by vitamins.

Weight Control

Be not a twiggy nor a piggy!

Most medical experts agree that being extremely underweight or very overweight is unhealthy. Women who are underweight have osteoporosis more often than overweight women. Remember that weight goals should be individual and personal, determined with your doctor in relation to your existing state of health, your own weight history, and how your weight is proportioned between lean body tissues and fat. Weight charts are being revised upward after many studies have shown that people with average or slightly above average weight live the longest. And weight control is more a permanent way of eating, modifying food habits, rather than quickie diets. (For tables of desirable weights for adults, refer to the booklet *Eating for Health*, D.H.S.S., from Her Majesty's Stationery Office.)

Dieting. Are you constantly going on the latest slimming diet or food fad? If you are always dieting – trying to lose those last 5 pounds – you may also be losing bone as well as body fat.

So many people are swayed by diet writers who like to link slimness with beauty, glamour, success and high fashion. The fashion industry has a lot to answer for, in encouraging women to be emaciated and, literally, bone-thin.

Food fads and regimens sweep the country from time to time, promising to take off weight rapidly, with no effort by the dieter; but most have serious drawbacks, limiting food selections, cutting out some essential nutrients, and reducing calcium and vitamins to dangerously low levels. Some diets emphasize individual foods or single food groups, like the banana diet and grapefruit diet, but no food is complete in its nutrition, and if eaten exclusively it can cause other deficiencies.

Low-calorie liquid diets have been popular, but should be undertaken under a doctor's supervision for a short time only, since they are usually low in potassium and can cause heart abnormalities.

High-fibre weight-loss diets are frequently low in calcium, with dairy products under-emphasized or entirely eliminated. These diets allow large amounts of food to be eaten, but are excessively high in fibre or include a tablespoon of mineral oil or liquid paraffin at each meal; thus the nutrients in food are prevented from being absorbed while passing through the intestine, with the result that vitamins and minerals such as calcium also pass through without absorption into your body. (For more on dietary fibre, see the 'Laxatives' section on p. 44.)

Diet pills (anorectics), either on prescription or over-the-counter products, that suppress the appetite have been popular as a quick way to lose weight. They generally deaden the sense of taste and the appetite, but at the same time they can increase blood pressure and metabolism. Prescription anorectics are mostly amphetamines or similar drugs, with the side effects of insomnia, nervousness, palpitations, increased pulse rate, higher blood pressure, dry mouth, diarrhoea and depression. Over a length of time you can become addicted to them.

Some women use diuretics as an aid to (temporary) weight-loss, but by increasing urine, these pills also increase loss of calcium.

Few low-calorie diets have the necessary amounts of calcium to maintain bone tissue – and it is especially dangerous for young girls who attempt fasting as they are consuming no calcium at all. Extensive fasting for religious beliefs or extremist political reasons can be equally hazardous.

First ask yourself if you *really* are overweight. Diet specialists realize that weight control is an interplay between our society's culture and mass psychology, with personal psychology and physiology. Weight control is based on a simple formula: the number of calories taken in, minus the number of calories expended should equal zero or a minus figure. To lose weight, consume fewer calories with smaller portions (especially fats, sugar and starchy foods, and alcohol), and exercise more to speed metabolism, and actually decrease appetite. Decreasing calories to around 1200 or 1500 a day, choosing foods from the four basic food groups, with *some* fibre for bulk, plus increasing exercise, can help you lose poundage. Whole food in its naturally unprocessed state is generally lower calorie. But even though calorie-poor, make sure you are calcium-rich, with foods such as skimmed milk, lowfat cheese, yogurt and buttermilk. Discuss calcium supplements with your doctor or a dietician.

Children and teenagers should not go on diets until after their growth period has finished, unless under close medical supervision, as muscles and bone mass are still developing. Similarly, it is not advisable for pregnant women to undertake diets unless under the direction of their personal physician. Most doctors believe the proper weight gain during pregnancy should be between 22 and 35 pounds (10–16kg). It would be better for breast-feeding mothers who are anxious to lose their prenatal weight gain to do so slowly until they have finished breast feeding, otherwise their milk supply will suffer or their own skeletal calcium reserves will be depleted.

Anorexia Nervosa. This disorder (after the Greek 'anorexis', without longing, without appetite) is dieting to the point of self-starvation, with an obsessive desire to be ultra thin, because of peer pressure among young women or the power of advertising. A girl with this condition can literally waste away to death. It is not well known in countries where there are *real* shortages of food, but it seems to be on the increase in the Western world where it mainly affects young girls. Recent conservative estimates indicate that 1 in 100 schoolgirls in Britain have anorexia to some degree. Although most anorexics are female, about 6 per cent are adolescent boys; occasionally the disorder is found in older women.

An anorexic may begin to diet to lose a few pounds, but become so intent on losing weight, with a revulsion towards food, she starves herself until weighing perhaps only 60 or 70 pounds – while still falsely believing herself to be fat.

Hormonal changes occur to make her reproductive system unbalanced, she will become infertile and cease to menstruate because of oestrogen deficiency, she will risk heart failure, kidney failure and liver damage. Nutrition has no chance to build up her bone structure, and with frequent induced vomiting, her teeth decay rapidly with the bile acids that rot the enamel.

Researchers at Massachusetts General Hospital report that although most of the damaging consequences of anorexia nervosa are reversible with therapy and weight gain, the reduction in bone density might not be. Bone building may resume with a return to normal eating habits, but it may be impossible to compensate for the time when bone growth was impaired.

Reduced bone mass may continue throughout the lives of formerly anorexic girls, making them even more vulnerable to postmenopausal fracturing.

To effect a cure, counselling and individual therapy is vital, if you have a daughter with this disorder, or know a young person on a deliberate starvation diet.

Bulimia. This disorder (from the Greek for 'ox hunger') concerning excessive eating, is a related form of anorexia nervosa. Bulimia was known in Roman times, but appears to have been re-invented in the last few years, or perhaps it is just coming out into the open. In 1980 it was listed as a formal psychiatric diagnosis by the American Psychiatric Association.

People with this illness go on 'food binges' and then purge themselves immediately after eating, through vomiting (often induced with Ipecac) or through the heavy use of laxatives or diuretics. With this disorder, the intestines have a reduced chance of absorbing nutrients from food intake.

Anorexia and bulimia affect approximately 5 per cent of the population, especially young women, with bulimia the more common disorder. Treatment for the problem needs the help of doctors, therapists and nutritionists for counselling.

Obesity. It's a good idea to keep weight constant, as already-weakened bones may not be capable of supporting an extra 20 or 30 pounds.

In the 1983 report *Obesity* by the Royal College of Physicians, 8 per cent of women and 6 per cent of men are obese. Chronically overweight women seldom suffer from osteoporosis, probably because they put heavier stress on their bones, with the bone responding by building new tissue to meet the demand for more strength. Or it could be that larger women produce more of the male hormone, androgen, which in turn is converted to oestrogen to reduce the risk of bone loss.

Because of this higher production of androgen hormones after menopause, being obese (or grossly overweight) increases the chances of endometrial cancer (cancer of the lining of the uterus). Obesity also increases the risk of cancers of the cervix, uterus, ovaries and breast, and of developing high blood pressure, heart disease and diabetes.

If you are seriously overweight, ask your doctor to refer you to a trained dietician for expert advice.

Laxatives

According to D.H.S.S. estimates for 1987, the ingredients for prescription laxatives and purgatives cost £12.5 million, with more millions spent on non-prescription aids. As many as 22 per cent of people in Britain admit to taking laxatives regularly – many are not needed, some are harmful and possibly habit-forming. The frequent and excessive use of laxatives may lead to bone depletion, by stimulating the passage of food too quickly through the intestinal tract before nutrients are absorbed. Or laxatives can give the feeling of fulness that reduces appetite, leading to a reduction in your intake of nourishing food.

There is overuse of mineral oil or liquid paraffin, widely used in nursing homes and by the elderly: as little as 4 teaspoons of mineral oil twice daily is sufficient to reduce the absorption of vitamins A, D, E and K and can also cause side effects with other drugs.

While fibre in your diet can be a blessing for relieving constipation, preventing diverticulitis and lowering blood cholesterol, too much bran fibre can be detrimental, increasing your loss of calcium, phosphorus, magnesium, iron and zinc. The bran from the outer husks of cereals such as wheat and oats contains phytates that interfere with calcium absorption.

Alpha cellulose (wood pulp or finely-ground sawdust) has lately been added by some food manufacturers to bread, rolls and biscuits, to increase fibre content. But wood pulp fibre has no nutritive value, and no one knows what the long-range effects of eating it will be. There could be loss of essential nutrients if you are eating many foods containing cellulose at the expense of good nutrition from other foods.

Ask yourself if you *really* are constipated. 'Regularity' can be defined as perhaps a twice-daily bowel movement for some people, and twice-weekly for others. Know what is 'normal' for you, to avoid laxative dependence. Doctors agree that constipation is frequently overemphasized, fostered by the manufacturers of laxative products, and older people become too concerned with the importance of having a bowel movement each day. This is a myth. Another fallacy is that wastes stored in the body are absorbed, are dangerous to health, or shorten life span. The huge sales of laxatives are based on these false beliefs.

But if you are unused to taking large quantities of milk or calcium supplements, they can be constipating, as can drugs such as pain medications, antidepressants, antacids containing aluminium or calcium, antihistamines, diuretics, anti-Parkinsonism drugs, anticonvulsants for epilepsy and iron supplements. Travel, prolonged bed-rest and certain hormonal disturbances such as an underactive thyroid gland can produce constipation, and it is well known that pregnancy can cause it. Injuries to the spinal cord and tumours pressing on the spinal cord may produce constipation by affecting the nerves that lead to the intestine.

To tone up your system without using harsh laxatives, try to get more exercise, more liquids (unless suffering from certain kidney or heart diseases), and a change in diet. Avoid the heavy use of convenience foods or soft processed foods that are low in fibre.

High-fibre food should be a necessary part of your daily meals, but used in moderation without going to extremes, as excessive quantities can cause harm, by putting you at risk of poor mineral absorption. How much dietary fibre we each need is still not certain, and estimates range between 25 and 50 grams per day. An ideal amount allows for proper absorption of minerals, vitamins and other food nutrients, while giving normal bowel movements. Although meat may *look* fibrous, dietary fibre is found in foodstuffs from plants and *not* from animals – preferably from generous portions of whole fruits (including skins), vegetables, legumes (beans and peas, for instance) and wholewheat breads rather than bran. There are about 9 grams of fibre in ½ cup serving of beans or peas; about 5 grams of fibre in ½ to ¾ cup of cooked vegetables or 1 oz (30 g) of raw nuts; about 3 grams of fibre in a medium-sized fruit, in 2 tablespoons of wholegrain breakfast cereals or two slices of wholewheat bread.

The benefit of vegetarianism

There are many reasons why some people choose to adopt vegetarianism: sometimes it is because meat is hard to obtain or too expensive; it may be due to religious beliefs, objections to killing animals or a fear of chemicals used to fatten livestock; it may be as a political protest against 'agribusiness'; some people may simply not care for the taste of meat, or find it difficult to chew with poor teeth. For whatever reason, vegetarianism is becoming increasingly popular, with several supermarket chains and major restaurants catering to the bigger demand for healthy meatless meals.

While care should be taken to avoid deficiencies in certain nutrients, studies of lacto-ovo-vegetarians indicate they have only about half the bone loss of meat-eaters, so the inference is that a high intake of protein from meats may contribute to bone loss. (The problem of high protein intake is covered in the next section.)

Strictly speaking, a *vegetarian* is a person who refuses to eat meat, poultry or fish. A *lacto-vegetarian* allows dairy products and an *ovo-vegetarian* permits eggs; a *lacto-ovo-vegetarian* eats both milk products and eggs. The most liberal vegetarians are those who eat fish, poultry, eggs and dairy products, fruits and vegetables, but exclude the red meats (beef, lamb or pork).

However, some vegetarianism is more extreme – and the more restrictions are observed, the greater the potential for general undernutrition: a *fruitarian* is limited to only raw or dried fruits, nuts and sometimes honey. A *vegan* or *strict vegetarian* eats only plant food, no animal flesh nor other animal food such as eggs or dairy products. These diets are usually low in calcium and vitamin D when dairy products are not eaten, and the loss is not made up by other sources of calcium found in vegetables. When vegan mothers breast-feed their babies, some cases of rickets (osteomalacia) have occurred, so many are now turning to soya milk that has been fortified with calcium and vitamins.

One of the most restrictive diets is the Zen *macrobiotic* system of cereals, soups, and hardly any fruits, with a restriction of fluids. Over a period of time, such severe diets can lead to scurvy, anaemia, protein deficiency, loss of kidney function, loss of calcium, with severe bone reduction and emaciation. A recent study in Boston found that growth was retarded in a group of children consuming a strict macrobiotic diet.

For handy guides to healthy meatless eating, read *The New Vegetarian* by Michael Cox and Desda Crockett (Thorsons), and *The Best of Vegetarian Cooking* by Janet Hunt (Thorsons).

Too much protein

Protein is one of the building-blocks in your body, a vital daily nutrient needed among other things, for the formation of new tissue, the production of antibodies to resist infections and for normal blood clotting. Osteoporosis can develop from either a lack of protein or too much.

In the average British diet, 66 per cent of protein comes from animal sources and 33 per cent is derived from plants. Most people are brought up believing that plenty of protein builds strong bones, whereas studies indicate that vegetarians (particularly those eating eggs and dairy products) have denser bones. While children, pregnant women, athletes and convalescents under the care of dieticians have special requirements for daily protein, people on average eat *twice* as much protein as they really need. Large quantities can be harmful, accelerating extensive calcium loss in the urine, particularly in osteoporotic women or those at risk of developing it in later years.

Excess protein puts a strain on the kidneys, increases body fat, and makes your body lose calcium, weakening bones and tooth-supporting tissue. Absorption of calcium seems to be best when protein intake is moderate: for a moderately active woman, no less than the World Health Organization recommendation of 29 grams of protein, and no more than the D.H.S.S. recommendation of 54 grams of protein per day.

In a study at Creighton University, Nebraska, a group of women each with an average protein intake of 50 per cent more than the recommended amount had an increased daily loss of calcium in their urine – a deficit leading to an annual loss rate of 1 per cent of their bone mass.

Protein is found mostly in meats, poultry, fish and dairy products – but don't cut back on dairy products as they are important sources of calcium. Many health experts suggest that, if you eat meat, have it no more than three times a week and keep portions small. By having hearty savoury casseroles of vegetable protein combinations, not only will you be counteracting bone loss, you'll be increasing fibre and reducing intake of fats and phosphorus. (See 'Calcium to phosphorus ratio' in chapter 5.)

What contraceptive do you use?

The Pill is associated with risks of high blood pressure, blood clotting (thrombosis), and cardiovascular disease; but evidence suggests stronger bones for women who have used the Pill for extensive periods of time. The positive effect on bones is related to the amounts of oestrogen and progestogen in the oral contraceptives, with these hormones also probably stimulating the release of calcitonin to inhibit bone reduction. The Pill may maintain or strengthen your bone mass.

But even the new oral contraceptives are not risk-free, and they can interact with other drugs you may be taking, altering their effectiveness – certain antibiotics, epilepsy drugs, anti-inflammatory or anti-arthritic drugs and barbiturates, for instance. Your doctor will probably only prescribe them if you –

● are under the age of thirty-five,
● do not smoke,
● have normal or low blood pressure and normal cholesterol level,
● are no more than 30 per cent overweight,
● have never had diabetes, liver or gallbladder disease; cancer of the liver, breast or reproductive tract (uterus, ovaries or cervix); epilepsy, migraine headaches, or exposure to DES (Diethylstilbesterol) before you were born.

Read the 'patient leaflet' that usually comes with oral contraceptives. They tend to change your body chemistry and the use your body makes of food nutrients. Consequently you may have a deficiency in vitamin B_6, vitamin C and folic acid that you will need to make up with generous servings of orange juice, wholegrain breads and green vegetables daily.

How soon to have children, and how many?

During pregnancy there is usually a natural high level of oestrogen to promote the production of active vitamin D, encouraging calcium absorption. There are also much higher levels of progesterone during pregnancy, to conserve the bone mass. Therefore pregnancy can be beneficial to your bone mass if your daily consumption of calcium is adequate for your body and for the formation of your unborn baby. The conclusion among many doctors is that if you have *not* had children, your risk of osteoporosis may be higher.

If, on the other hand, a teenager becomes pregnant before her bone mass has reached skeletal maturity (in 1982, 90,000 teenagers in England and Wales were pregnant), and if an expectant or nursing mother does not maintain an adequate daily intake of calcium, or embarks on unwise dieting before lactation is finished, her body will steal from its own skeletal reserves to nourish the foetus and provide lactation. This explains the origin of the old saying 'for every child, a tooth'.

Similarly, in poor countries where the level of nutrition is low, pregnancy and a lengthy period of breast-feeding can have a debilitating effect on a mother's skeleton. Whatever calcium is available goes straight to the foetus to start bone building. With an insufficient intake, the mother's calcium reserves in her skeleton will be drawn upon.

A new type of woman is becoming pregnant today – the older career woman who decides to have a family at a later date in her life. She may already be at an age when she is starting to lose trabecular bone tissue from her vertebrae, making good nutrition of vital importance, and sufficient intake of calcium essential.

If you have many pregnancies at frequent intervals, with no due regard to proper nutrition, each child will represent a drain on your calcium reserves and bone strength.

Many experts consider it prudent to build up calcium levels *before* pregnancy.

Do you smoke?

Studies are continuing on the links between smoking and osteoporosis, and certain facts are known.

Women are starting to smoke at a younger age, frequently to stay on diets. Smokers are more likely to be underweight. Pregnant mothers who smoke have babies that are on average 200 grams smaller than babies whose mothers do not. Oestrogen levels are lower in smokers, and they have menopause at an earlier age, hastening it by as much as five years, exposing them to greater risk. Studies of groups of osteoporotic women revealed that over 75 per cent were smokers, and more than 66 per cent smoked more than a pack of cigarettes a day. It has been speculated that there may be a relationship between smoking and the effective functioning of the liver where vitamin D is activated. If smoking impedes the system of the activation of vitamin D, less calcium is absorbed, creating a calcium deficit and subsequent bone loss.

According to a report from the Office of Population Censuses and Surveys (General Household Survey 1988), 32 per cent of people in Britain are smokers, and of this number, 52 per cent are women. Furthermore, women were smoking more cigarettes per week in 1984 than in 1972. 25 per cent of girls were smoking by the age of sixteen, compared with 16 per cent of boys. Medical authorities consider the age at which you start to smoke is crucial, because the earlier you begin, the longer is your exposure to tobacco and the risk of smoking-related illnesses, such as lung cancer, heart disease, chronic bronchitis and emphysema. *Smoking is deadly!*

The British Medical Association is now urging the phasing out of all advertising and promotion of tobacco products, and stressing the printing of sterner health warnings on cigarette packets. In the United States, most states have laws banning smoking in public buildings, restrictions in factories and shops, and many restaurants have 'No smoking' sections. Unfortunately, cigarette manufacturers try to equate smoking with Women's Liberation or project cigarettes as part of a glamorous style young people should copy.

According to a study completed recently by the US Environmental Protection Agency, chronic exposure to tobacco smoke can also affect *non*-smokers to the same extent as smoking one to ten cigarettes a day.

Some young people are turning to 'alternative' choices of clove cigarettes (kreteks) or chewing tobacco, as the newest fads. Clove cigarettes, imported from Indonesia, are often labelled as a herbal low-tobacco substitute, but laboratory analysis shows their composition to be 60 per cent tobacco and 40 per cent cloves. Studies indicate that they are in no way a safe substitute for conventional cigarettes. Because clove cigarettes are unfiltered, they produce almost twice as much tar, nicotine and carbon monoxide as ordinary moderate-tar cigarettes, and have associated risks of nosebleeds, lung infections and asthma. 30 per cent of clove cigarette smokers cough up blood. Eugenol is a major component of cloves and, while it is recognized as safe when eaten as a spice in foods, evidence has shown eugenol to be unsafe for inhaling. This has prompted the American Lung Association and the American Health Foundation to issue stern warnings about the danger of clove cigarette use.

Chewing tobacco and snuff have a direct relationship with the development of cancer of the gums and mouth. According to an Ohio journal *Preventive Medicine Monthly* (November 1984), smokeless tobacco can cause 'discolored teeth and fillings, destruction of periodontal bond and soft tissue, slow-healing cuts and sores in the mouth and increased tooth sensitivity . . . The habit may also cause gums to recede, teeth to become vulnerable, drift from position and fall out . . .'.

The time to quit is now! Many smokers can stop easily, but most have difficulty even though well-motivated. Some smokers find it beneficial to join groups in cigarette-withdrawal clinics. Others can fight nicotine addiction with various products available at the chemist.

For instance, some smokers find nicotine chewing gum is effective. 'Nicorette' is a prescription drug in chewing gum form, used as a temporary crutch for smokers trying to stop, especially in programmes supervised by doctors or in stop-smoking groups or clinics. The patented formulation is made in Denmark by A. B. Leo, a Swedish company, and at the moment it is the only brand on the world market, available in the UK, USA, Europe, Canada and Australia. The nicotine in this gum is absorbed through the lining of the mouth directly into the bloodstream. Overall blood levels of nicotine are similar to those obtained from cigarettes, the rate of release of nicotine being controlled by the rate of chewing. The object is to relieve withdrawal symptoms of a smoker; the smoker still has to adjust to living without cigarettes. Check with your dentist before using 'Nicorette' as up to 2 per cent of users report dislodged dental fillings, loosened inlays and gummed-up dentures.

Another smoking-deterrent chewing gum containing silver acetate is available at chemists without a prescription, under the brand name 'Tabmint'. This product works differently, producing an unpleasant metallic taste in your mouth if you attempt to smoke while chewing the gum. This nasty effect can last for up to four hours, making smoking less desirable. Study results vary, but the product does appear to reduce or stop the use of cigarettes over a few weeks' time. The US Food and Drug Administration has established the safety of silver acetate gum when used for no longer than three weeks. If used excessively, it may cause permanent bluish-grey discoloration in your mouth. You should not use it when pregnant, and it should be kept away from children.

Among other products to help stop smoking are 'Test 60' tablets by Ashe Laboratories and 'Nicobrevin' capsules made in West Germany. A variety of filters can be attached to a cigarette, reducing tar and nicotine inhaled, but they have not been effective in assisting smokers to stop.

Do you take alcohol?

Although insufficient information is available on whether *moderate* amounts of alcohol have an effect on bone loss, it has been observed that heavy drinkers have abnormally light bones that fracture easily, with impairment of calcium absorption through the intestines. Alcoholism produces inflammation of the liver, causing damaged cells to be replaced by scar tissue that impairs the organ's function. Thus there is a reduced ability to produce enzymes for digestion and absorption of food nutrients.

Male alcoholics in their twenties have been known to have osteoporosis. A research team from Loma Linda University and Jerry Pettis Veterans Administration Hospital in California, has evidence that alcohol itself accelerates the breakdown of bone, although it is still uncertain whether alcoholics' bone problems may also be the results of poor diet, the inability of the liver to activate vitamin D, and/or a lack of exercise. Heavy drinkers may be taking certain antacids to soothe their stomachs, adding further to their bone problems.

It is the amount of alcohol you drink, and not the particular kind of drink that the alcohol is in. Thus 1½ oz of whisky equals

6 oz of wine, equals 12 oz of beer. Pure alcohol is 200° proof. Distilled spirits such as brandy, gin, vodka and whisky are about 40 per cent alcohol (80° proof). Fortified wines such as port, Madeira and sherry are about 20 per cent alcohol. Table wines, whether light or full-bodied, are about 10 per cent alcohol. Beers are about 5 per cent alcohol.

Many medications contain alcohol – for instance, medicines for coughs, colds and congestion – because alcohol is a better solvent and provides longer shelf-life than a water solution. A concentration of alcohol up to 35 per cent is used in many mouthwashes.

The problem is that we don't stop to consider that alcoholic beverages are drugs that can have interactions with many other drugs, both over-the-counter and prescription. Alcohol can cause other drugs to be used more rapidly by your body, producing exaggerated effects (mixing alcohol with a high dosage of 'Valium' or 'Darvon' can be fatal). Drugs can intensify your reaction to alcohol, leading to more rapid intoxication. Your body's response can also be influenced by menstrual periods and hormone levels, including the taking of oral contraceptives or hormone replacements after menopause – slowing the rate at which alcohol clears from your bloodstream.

Two-thirds of the population drink alcohol and certainly don't think of themselves as drug users. Alcohol is present at most of the big celebrations: births and christenings, birthdays, graduations, weddings, promotions, deaths and funerals. Holidays and Christmas revolve around having a drink with family and friends.

But ask yourself honestly if you are drinking more than a moderate amount each day – an important factor when considering loss of bone mass. How would you answer the following questions?

- Have you lost interest in food?
- Do you crave a drink at a definite time each day, and need to drink more to get the desired effect?
- Do you drink to put yourself to sleep?
- Do you gulp drinks too fast?
- Do you drink alone?
- Do you drink because you are shy, need to calm your nerves or bolster your confidence?

- Do you lie about how much you drink – and feel guilty?
- Are you losing time from work because of drinking?
- Has your efficiency and ambition decreased because of drinking?
- Has drinking made you indifferent about your family?
- Do you drink to forget problems at home, at work, or to reduce depression?
- Is drinking making your life at home unhappy?
- Are you in financial trouble because of heavy drinking?
- Have you sought the help of a doctor or been to hospital because of drinking?

Although alcohol abuse has been closely linked to the stresses of old age, with some studies estimating that 10 per cent to 15 per cent of people over the age of fifty-five may have a drinking problem, there is also great concern for the epidemic of teenage drinking. But the teen years are when the body should be building up its skeletal mass at the average rate of 10 per cent a year. Some young people under eighteen are already alcoholics or nearly so; many more are heading towards problem drinking that may be a lifetime handicap. Discourage your young daughter from drinking and smoking, and set yourself as an example.

For control of alcoholic beverage consumption, a physician will sometimes prescribe disulfiram ('Antabuse' by C. P. Pharmaceuticals) which is formulated to cause palpitations, flushing, sweating, shortness of breath or dizziness when even a small amount of drink is consumed or other drugs containing alcohol are taken.

Stress
Whether the stress is physical or emotional, it stimulates the adrenal hormones that cause bone depletion and much calcium can be lost in the urine. Stress may also reduce the amount of calcium absorbed by the intestines and maintained in your skeleton. It can also increase cholesterol in the bloodstream, acid in the stomach, and depress your immune system so your body's resistance to viruses and infections is lowered. But studies have not yet revealed why, in similar situations, some people seem almost stress-proof and others are highly vulnerable.

Nobody lives in a stress-free world. We all have stress –
anxiety, grief, boredom. But to rid our lives of all problems would
be the biggest problem of all. Normal stress is good, helping us to
cope with life, with sudden emergencies, and to adapt to change.
But excess stress can be *distress*.

Don't rush to take a pill: try different ways to manage your
emotions:

Try to relax – listen to music – read a good book.

Try recreation with friends – take regular holidays.

Try expressing your emotions – talk to someone to share
problems.

Try meditation.

Try some form of relaxing exercise – go for a walk.

Or accept the situation that is creating the stress. If you realize
you've been pushing yourself too hard, ease off the pressure.

Do you have indigestion?

With women playing a larger role today in positions of greater
responsibility and decision-making in business, or in stressful
situations managing a home (perhaps without a spouse), their
systems can react with problems of indigestion or ulcers. The
D.H.S.S. estimates for 1987 that the ingredients for prescription
antacids cost £20.9 million, with millions more spent on non-
prescription indigestion remedies. Growing numbers of women
are consuming them on a regular basis without knowing the
potential risk.

Many aids to digestion contain *aluminium* and some have
calcium in their ingredients. Which type you choose could be
important to your bone mass. When antacids contain aluminium,
extra calcium is excreted, with the calcium coming from your
bones. A side effect is constipation, but the greatest concern to
bone specialists is the aluminium (even in small amounts) that
combines with dietary phosphorus and calcium, drawing them out
of your body into the urine, thus probably weakening bones and
leading to osteoporosis and osteomalacia.

It's better to alter your meals and/or lifestyle to reduce your
indigestion problems without resorting to antacids. But if that is
not possible, at least change to an antacid without aluminium. If

you are at risk of osteoporosis, indigestion remedies containing calcium would be good substitutes, neutralizing acid and serving as a calcium supplement as well. Examine the labels carefully on antacid boxes and jars, or seek the help of the chemist or your doctor.

Speaking in Manchester at the 1985 Congress of the International Union of Pure and Applied Chemistry, Professor John Savory, pathologist, said 'Aluminium toxicity is the most important trace metal related to bone disease.'

In this aluminium-using society, there are other ways the substance can enter our bodies:

- It is in drinking water clarified by adding alum powder or aluminium salts (a problem in the North of England, e.g., Stockport and Newcastle, where towns are supplied with water from Pennine reservoirs). Aluminium may also be in drinking water after acid rain has leaked trace amounts of the metal from clay soils into water supplies. Ask your local Water Authority for the aluminium content of the tap water you use for drinking and cooking. If it is high, change to bottled water.
- It is absorbed into the skin from some underarm deodorants.
- It is added to many foods (household baking powders, individually-wrapped processed cheeses, pancake mixes, frozen dough, some pickled cucumbers, glacé cherries, and 'silver' dragees for cake decorating).
- Aluminium cookware can add to your daily intake if pans are old and worn, especially when salty, acidic or alkaline foods are cooked in them. It would be prudent to look critically at your aluminium saucepans and discard any with pitted surfaces.
- Do not use aluminium pellets when weighting the pastry of flans – substitute ceramic or glass beads or dry beans.

Do you use diuretics?

In cases of high blood pressure, doctors frequently prescribe diuretics to decrease water retention and increase the release of urine. In 1984 doctors issued over 5 million prescriptions for thiazide and over 4 million for furosemide. Discuss your prescription with your doctor, as a furosemide-type diuretic increases calcium excretion in the urine, while thiazides reduce calcium loss and would be preferable in many cases.

Diuretics are sometimes purchased as over-the-counter remedies to counter water retention, and many women abuse them with excessive use in order to lose weight (temporarily).

If your water retention is a monthly occurrence as a premenstrual condition, it can frequently be controlled by a saltless or sodium-free diet in the week immediately before your menstrual period, and by eating naturally-diuretic foods such as bananas, oranges, apples, cucumbers, strawberries, grapes and pineapple.

Salt and sodium

Ordinary table salt is sodium chloride, and sodium is very necessary for us. Sodium attracts water into the blood vessels, keeping the proper blood volume and the pressure within the blood vessels more or less constant, regulated by your kidneys. But, as you probably know, too much salt is unhealthy, increasing blood pressure and the risk of heart disease and kidney problems, and many of us consume salt in far greater quantities than necessary. A high intake of sodium can also lead to an extraction of calcium into the urine, although at the moment it is uncertain what is an excessive amount. But the conservative approach is to maintain a low-salt diet – no more than 2000 mg per day, as recommended by the World Health Organization and the American Heart Association.

Apart from table salt, sodium is found in many other foods, naturally present or as a part of processing and preserving. The wisest course is to eat fresh unprocessed foods as much as possible, seasoning generously with herbs and spices. When eating out, forsake fast foods and choose the salad bar without a large serving of dressing. Table 1 gives a brief list of sodium in foods. For more on this subject of reducing salt and sodium, see *The Salt-Watcher's Guide: Easy Ways to Cut Down on Salt and Sodium* by Kathleen Mayes (Thorsons, 1986).

Table 1

The Sodium Content of Your Food

Item	Sodium (mg)
Beverages (Alcoholic)	
Beer, draught bitter, ½ pt	33
White wine, 4 fl oz	21
Beverages (Non-alcoholic)	
Bournvita, 2 tbsp	69
Coca-Cola, 4 fl oz	8
Cocoa powder, 2 tbsp	142
Lucozade, 4 fl oz	30
Soda water, 4 fl oz	28
Tomato juice, canned, 4 fl oz	240
Dairy Products	
Cheeses:	
Cottage, 100 g/3½ oz	450
Danish Blue, 25 g/1 oz	355
Parmesan, 25 g/1 oz	190
Processed, 25 g/1 oz	340
Roquefort, 25 g/1 oz	458
Milk, whole, ½ pt	150
Malted milk, 2 tbsp	49
Yogurt, natural, 100 g/3½ oz	76
Eggs, Fish, Meat	
Corned beef, canned, 85 g/3 oz	807
Egg, whole, 1 egg	70
Ham, 85 g/3 oz	1062
Herring, pickled, 85 g/3 oz	1445
Pork pie, 100 g/3½ oz	720
Salmon, canned, 85 g/3 oz	484
Sausage, beef, 85 g/3 oz	935
Tuna, canned, 85 g/3 oz	357
Veal, jellied, canned, 85 g/3 oz	1011

Item	Sodium (mg)
Fats, Margarines, Oils	
Butter, salted, 25 g/1 oz	217
Low-fat spread, 15 g/1 tbsp	103
Margarine, salted, 15 g/1 tbsp	120
Vegetable oil, 15 g/1 tbsp	Tr.
Fruits	
Apple, 1 medium	2
Avocado	4
Banana, 1 medium	1
Grapes, 10 grapes	1
Orange, whole	2
Grain products	
Biscuits, semi-sweet, 25 g/1 oz	102
Bread, Hovis, 25 g/1 oz	145
Bread, soda, 25 g/1 oz	102
Breakfast cereals:	
All-Bran, 25 g/1 oz	382
Muesli, commercial, 25 g/1 oz	45
Shredded Wheat, 25 g/1 oz	3
Cakes:	
Ginger, commercial, 50 g/2 oz	245
Madeira, 50 g/2 oz	190
Swiss-roll, commercial, 50 g/2 oz	210
Spaghetti, canned, 100 g/3½ oz	500
Legumes	
Beans, baked, 100 g/3½ oz	480
Beans, kidney, 100 g/3½ oz	40
Soya beans, tofu, 100 g/3½ oz	7

Item	Sodium (mg)	Item	Sodium (mg)
Nuts		Potatoes, instant, 100 g/3½ oz	1190
Almonds, salted, 100 g/3½ oz	198	Sweetcorn, canned,	
Peanuts, salted, 100 g/3½ oz	440	100 g/3½ oz	310
		Tomato, raw	4
Soups		Tomato sauce (for cooking)	
Beef broth, canned, 1 cup	1224	100 g/3½ oz	850
Chicken noodle, 1 cup	888		
Oxtail, low-calorie, 1 cup	1248	*Condiments*	
		Garlic salt, 1 tsp	1456
Sugars and Sweets		Horseradish, prepared, 1 tbsp	60
Butterscotch, 25 g/1 oz	175	Mustard, English, prepared,	
Chocolate, milk, 25 g/1 oz	30	1 tbsp	510
		Olives, 4 green	562
Vegetables		Onion salt, 1 tsp	1455
Beans, French, canned,		Pickles, sweet, 1 tbsp	255
100 g/3½ oz	392	Salt, 1 tsp	1942
Beetroot, 100 g/3½ oz	64	Soya sauce, 1 tbsp	1468
Carrots, canned, 100 g/3½ oz	280	Worcestershire sauce, 1 tbsp	195
Peas, canned, 100 g/3½ oz	230		

Is your water supply 'hard' or 'soft'?

Do you think your local water feels 'hard' or 'soft'? Check the mineral content with your water company or local health authority. Where water flows over granite or other impervious rocks, few minerals are dissolved, and the water is often referred to as 'soft'. Thus, although the water feels good for bathing and makes laundry easier, there are fewer trace elements going into the water you drink. 'Soft' water can therefore have a range of about 10 to 30 mg of calcium per quart (litre).

If, on the other hand, the water seems 'hard', it might be giving you up to 100 mg of calcium per quart (litre), in those dissolved minerals. If you decide to have a household water softener, or a water-purifying system for drinking water, remember that such systems can remove valuable calcium as well as magnesium from the water. Check with your dealer. Softeners may also increase the sodium content of water by up to 300 mg per quart (litre), so drinking softened water is not recommended.

Fluoride

In water supplies. Fluorides are chemical combinations of fluorine and other common elements. Fluoride is an important mineral needed for good bones, blood, teeth, nails, skin and hair.

When fluoride is taken during childhood or adolescence, it is incorporated into the structure of developing teeth, making the enamel more resistant to acids produced by bacteria, as well as strengthening bone tissue. Fluoride is rapidly taken up by bone and is known to stimulate bone growth, and it has been used successfully in experiments treating sufferers of osteoporosis. Harvard studies have shown that elderly people suffer less calcium loss from bones and fewer hip fractures when fluoride is in their drinking water.

How much do you need? The US Recommended Daily Dietary Allowance for fluoride judged as safe and adequate has been established as follows:

Infants	0 to 6 months	0.1 to 0.5 mg
	6 months to 1 year	0.2 to 1.0 mg
Children	1 to 3 years	0.5 to 1.5 mg
	4 to 6 years	1.0 to 2.5 mg
	7 to 10 years	1.5 to 2.5 mg
	11 plus	1.5 to 2.5 mg
Adults		1.5 to 4.0 mg

Fluoride can occur naturally in water in certain localities, dissolving from rocks where the water is flowing. The optimum level is considered to be 1 part fluoride to a million parts of water (1 ppm), which provides a fluoride intake of about 1 milligram per day. Some regions have as little as 0.1 ppm and a few have as much as 5 to 10 ppm. The average level of natural fluoride in UK drinking water is low – only about 0.2 ppm. People who drink water containing higher levels of fluoride, such as 5 ppm, may have mottling of teeth but virtually no tooth decay and good strong bones. Moderate bone 'fluorosis' can be beneficial for greater skeletal strength among elderly people, and moderate fluoride supplements can prevent the onset of osteoporosis.

Too much fluoride can be as harmful as too little, however, although bone fluorosis generally occurs only where the fluoride level of water is more than 10 ppm (10 mg of fluoride per day). For instance, in the Punjab region of India, where the naturally present fluoride is extremely high, bone changes are connected with severe joint and nerve disease.

Fluoridation of public water supplies continues to create controversy, and perhaps you've heard about other possible adverse effects of fluoride. Fluoride *is* toxic at excessive levels, but 2500 ppm is required for fatal poisoning – many times higher than that in fluoridated water. And although you may hear rumours and reports that fluoride is associated with human cancer, there is no scientific truth or medical basis. Studies have tried to link fluoridated drinking water with Mongolism (Down's Syndrome), but have failed for lack of scientific evidence. The US Consumers Union medical panel has concluded that there is no scientific controversy over fluoridation safety, and finds it economical and beneficial.

Water Authorities in the UK have twenty-three different schemes for fluoridation of our water supplies, for about 9 million people or 17 per cent of the population. Check to see if your community water supply is naturally fluoridated, or if it has been amended to the approved level of 1 ppm of fluoride. If you have a reverse osmosis system in your home to provide purified drinking water, this could be removing fluoride. Check this with your dealer. And ask your physician or dentist about the fluoride needed by you and your family, and before giving fluoride tablets to your children.

Commercial companies that sell bottled drinking water some-times offer the option of water that has been treated with fluoride to the 1 ppm level, at a small extra cost compared to regular drinking water.

If your children are relying on fluoridated water as their source of fluoride, make sure they are actually drinking it, and not consuming the more tempting soft drinks.

Fluoride in foods. Although water is the main source of fluoride in the diet, it also occurs in various foods – sardines, whole fish, and tea, for instance. Food can contribute up to 25 per cent of your daily fluoride intake, particularly if fluoridated water is used in processing or the crops are grown in regions naturally high in fluoride. Tea leaves have the highest fluoride levels found in plants: 6 cups of an average brew in England supplies about 1 mg. A relatively high concentration of fluoride has been found in wine from grapes growing near active volcanoes in Italy. Table 2 gives a few examples of other foods. Note that as these figures for fluoride are in micrograms, the amounts are minute, but nonetheless important.

In other parts of the world, fluoride has been specially added to foods: in Hungary and Switzerland it has been added to salt. Experiments have also tried the fortification of fluoride in flour, milk, fruit juices and sugar.

Table 2
Fluoride in Foods

Food	Fluoride (micrograms/100g)	Food	Fluoride (micrograms/100g)
Almonds	90	Kale	16–300
Apples	5–130	Lamb	120
Cheese	160	Mackerel	2700
Chicken	140	Potatoes	7–640
Chocolate milk	50–200	Salmon, canned	450–900
Cod	700	Sardines, canned	730–1600
Coffee, instant	170	Shrimp, canned	440
Crab, canned	200	Tea	120–6300
Fishmeal	8000–25,000	Watercress	100
Herring, smoked	350	Wheat germ	88–400
Honey	100	Wine	0–630

How much coffee do you drink?

And how much is too much? When you have a cup of coffee, your body reacts to the caffeine by stimulating the nervous system, increasing heartbeat, basal metabolism and the secretion of stomach acid and an increase in urine. And studies have shown that heavy coffee-drinkers lose more calcium from their bodies than noncoffee-drinkers. As coffee may be a contributing factor in bone loss, it would be prudent to reduce consumption to no more than one cup a day. The key word is 'moderation'. Health authorities advise pregnant women to avoid caffeine altogether because studies indicate it could cause skeletal defects in unborn children. Other studies are now focused on the effects of caffeine on children because of the large quantities of soft drinks, iced tea and chocolate they may consume. The problem is that caffeine is not only in many drinks but also in many common foods and drugs, both prescription and non-prescription. Table 3 gives the latest scorecard on caffeine and illustrates its prevalence.

Caffeine in coffee and tea can vary because of different methods of brewing, and whether it is from standard ground beans, instant or decaffeinated. Black tea has high caffeine, green tea very low; completely caffeine-free teas have recently been introduced. The effect of caffeine in tea is less than in coffee because tea has other ingredients that slow down the release of caffeine. Lovers of chocolate can change to carob powder to avoid caffeine, reduce phosphorus and boost calcium.

Herbal teas have not yet been studied extensively in Britain, so if you drink herbal tea to avoid the known effects of caffeine, you could expose yourself to other chemicals about which far less is known. Although the vast majority of herbs are safe in normal amounts, you should not conclude that all herbal teas are safe, nor that it is safe to drink large amounts of any herbal teas, for a length of time.

Because of growing concern, an increasing number of soft drinks are now produced without caffeine, but they can be high in phosphorus. Read the labels on cans and bottles carefully.

Discuss caffeine with your doctor before taking any drugs, including simple over-the-counter medicines such as painkillers and sleeping preparations. Similar products without caffeine are usually available.

Table 3
Caffeine in Foods and Drinks

Item	Caffeine (mg)
Coffee, 5 oz cup:	
Brewed, drip	60–180
Brewed, percolator	40–170

Item	Caffeine (mg)
Coffee, 5oz cup:	
Instant	30–120
Tea, 5oz cup:	
Brewed	25–110
Instant	25–50
Cocoa beverage, 5oz cup	2–20
Chocolate milk beverage, 8oz	2–7
Chocolate bar, 1oz:	
Milk	1–15
Plain, semi-sweet	5–35
Baking chocolate	26
Soft drinks, 6oz:	
Regular colas	15–23
Decaffeinated colas	trace
Diet colas	1–29

(*Source: US Food and Drug Administration, Food Additive Evaluation Branch, March 1984*)

How much do you exercise?

Regular exercise is essential for maintaining muscle tone and putting stress on bones – necessary not only for halting bone loss but stimulating the formation of new stronger bone tissues.

Astronauts in space flights lost considerable amounts of bone tissue, at a rate of 0.5 per cent per month, after a short time in a weightless state. More recent missions have included exercise to try to prevent bone depletion; unfortunately, this exercise has proved ineffective without the stress and pull of gravity on bone and muscle.

Similar problems occur in hospital patients or those confined to wheelchairs – a condition called *disuse osteoporosis*. Bones weaken and shrink when not used, in a sedentary lifestyle, just as muscles do; bones respond by becoming stronger and larger when stress is placed on them with exercise. Exercise increases blood flow to bones, bringing in nutrients for new formation. Exercise can change the levels of the body's hormones that form bones, creating a better environment for new bone formation, increasing oestrogen and decreasing harmful adrenal hormones. When athletes build up muscles, the strenuous training also builds bone mass.

A study has been carried out at the University of North Carolina, Chapel Hill, USA, under the direction of orthopaedist Peter Jacobson: 400 sedentary women aged between thirty-five and sixty-five were compared with 80 women of the same age range who played tennis regularly each week. Of those under fifty-five, there were no special differences in bone structure. But women over fifty-five in the study had much stronger bones among the tennis-playing group. Research suggests that tennis, jogging and other 'weight-bearing' exercises may help to strengthen older bones.

Other studies of menopausal women have them square dancing, jazz dancing and performing isometrics to determine the changes in their bone mass. Bone loss may not be inevitable in later years, but proportional to a slowdown in exercise and physical activities.

Although many people think of themselves as being fairly active, very often their hectic lives mean they are mentally and socially active but not physically. Exercise is a Do-It-Yourself venture; no one else can do it for you. Make it a part of your lifestyle for the rest of your life!

At the same time you've got to strike the right balance: if you exercise as vigorously as some athletes that you stop menstruating, you can place yourself in danger of having bone loss as a result of lower oestrogen levels. Loss of menstruation, called *amenorrhoea*, occurs in up to 50 per cent of competitive runners and ballet dancers but affects only 3 to 5 per cent of women in general. If a woman does not menstruate for a year, she should have her bone density checked.

In recent research, Robert Marcus, M.D., of Stanford University School of Medicine, Christopher E. Cann, Ph.D., of University of California, San Francisco, and others, studied bone-mass variations in a group of white long-distance runners (running up to 160 kilometres a week). Of the seventeen women, six had regular menstrual periods and eleven had none. Four of the women without periods had started intense training before the onset of menses. The non-menstruating athletes had 17 per cent lower spine density than the menstruating women. Cortical bone mass was not apparently affected by lack of menstruation, but trabecular bone density was lower. The study supported the idea that intense physical training at an early age may delay menarche, and women would be better not to train to such an extent that they don't menstruate regularly.

Although athletes may be under pressure from coaches and peers to keep weight down, they still need to consume sufficient calories, calcium and protein, and avoid vitamin overdoses. Most importantly, non-menstruating athletes may need a greater intake of calcium daily, similar to postmenopausal women.

Women should not be frightened off exercise, however, as few have such tough multi-mile running programmes, as in the previously mentioned study, or do other aerobics so strenuously. The effect of regular exercise on bone density is positive, providing calcium intake is maintained; the benefits of exercise still far outweigh the hazards.

See more on exercise in chapter 7.

Taking care of your teeth

Periodontal disease can be either an indication of poor oral hygiene or a warning that underlying bone is becoming porous. It is often called gingivitis in its earlier stages, then periodontal disease as the condition advances, when tooth and bone loss may occur. The 1978 Adult Dental Health Survey reported that *91 per cent* of adults with their own teeth suffer in varying degrees with this disease of the gums and tooth-supporting tissues – conditions that can result in the loss of underlying alveolar bone containing the tooth sockets.

Mature teeth in an adult do not significantly change their structure or calcification with altered intakes of calcium or a change in calcium metabolism. Periodontal tissues, on the other hand, do have an active interchange of available nutrients similar to bone and soft tissues in other parts of the body. Dental researchers have concluded that insufficient calcium may contribute to the loss of alveolar bone and tooth-supporting tissues; there is also a strong connection between periodontal disease and the accumulation of plaque, the sticky semi-transparent material containing food debris, bacteria and toxins that irritate and destroy gum tissue and surrounding bone. Diseased or infected gums are often the cause of bad breath.

So there are two key points: (1) make sure you have adequate daily calcium in your food and (2) maintain good dental hygiene.

If plaque is not brushed off your teeth every day, it hardens into calculus (tartar) which can only be removed by your dentist or dental hygienist. Build-up of plaque and calculus can lead to gum disease, which if untreated can create pockets of infection. Eventually the structures that support the teeth are destroyed, the bony sockets around the roots of teeth begin to demineralize or resorb, and as the bone is lost, the teeth become loose and fall out. Good dental hygiene is the key to prevention of gum disease, with a programme of regular visits to your dentist.

Adults and teenagers should use fluoridated toothpastes and mouthwashes to help ward off dental decay and prevent gum disease. Some British toothpastes also have calcium in their formula to aid dental repair. It's vital to brush your teeth and gums with a soft toothbrush and floss daily to remove plaque the brush cannot reach. Fluoride in toothpaste works on the surface of teeth in two ways:

1. It stops the reproduction of *Streptococcus mutans*, the most powerful of many acid-making bacteria in your mouth. This bacterium feeds on the sugars and starches in your mouth and turns them into enamel-burning acid. *Streptococcus mutans* also is responsible for creating plaque, the gummy stuff that sticks to teeth to make a breeding spot for more bacteria; and

2. Fluoride allows the acid-scarred surface of teeth to heal. When fluoride is present in your mouth, calcium and phosphorus from saliva fill in the microscopic pits made by acid. Without fluoride, the pits get wider and deeper, and bacteria can penetrate further into the tooth enamel.

Cut down on sugar (all types: table sugar, fructose, maltose, glucose), sticky foods (like caramels, raisins, dates and soft drinks sweetened with sugar) and smoking. If you have mild periodontal disease, talk with your dentist about increasing your daily intake of calcium and vitamin C.

To maintain firm gums, healthy underlying bone and strong jaw muscles, give them sufficient *exercise* every day: let them go to work on crisp, crunchy fresh fruits and vegetables that need plenty of biting and chewing.

If you are already wearing dentures, make sure they are fitted properly and firmly – uniformly against the gums without uneven pressure on underlying bone. Brush your gums, ridges and palate with a soft brush to stimulate circulation, remove debris, and harden the tissue surface so that your dentures are most comfortable to wear.

Street drugs and drug abuse

Apart from the mind-bending and mind-scrambling, which is the attraction of street drugs, these substances and their impurities can have long-term complications that could have a bearing on bone mineralization.

The sniffing of *glues* and *aerosols* (aeroplane glue, plastic cements, paints, lacquers, thinners, cleaning fluids, petrol, lighter fuel) can damage the liver and kidneys. *Amphetamines* ('uppers') and *methamphetamines* ('speed') create loss of appetite down to starvation levels, leading to malnutrition. *Barbiturates* can cause an impairment of liver function, change metabolism, producing deficiencies of hormones and vitamins, and reducing calcium levels. Doctors report that girls and young women are now smoking *crack* or sniffing cocaine as a cheap and quick, but misguided, way to diet and lose weight. The drug reduces weight because it is an amphetamine and therefore an appetite suppressant, linked to eating disorders such as anorexia and bulimia. Young girls are being misled by drug dealers, who suggest crack to help lose pounds and get thin.

The Home Office reported that the number of registered drug addicts in Britain rose to 14,800 in 1989. Police claim that this figure should be multiplied by at least five to give a true indication of the number of addicts.

Not all drugs are illegally obtained; many women acquire them legally with doctors' prescriptions, perhaps without realizing they are becoming increasingly dependent on them.

Drug dependence will eventually cost you something in health, although not every drug abuser pays the same price for the same excess. Among heavy drug users, malnutrition is often the result of erratic and irregular meals, producing mineral and vitamin deficiencies. When the function of the liver is impaired, it may affect your ability to activate vitamin D, leading to a decreased absorption of calcium in your intestines.

With the right help, drug habits can be broken, although withdrawal can be painful and difficult, and it may take months. Getting off drugs can be done with outpatient or residential treatment, chemically-assisted or drug-free, depending on what programmes are available to you locally. Your family doctor may not be the ideal professional to talk to about turning off, and he may refer you to a specialist on drug dependency. Your health and local authorities have information about nearby help for drug-abuse. Or you can write to: The Institute for the Study of Drug Dependence, 1–4 Hatton Place, London, EC1N 8ND; or to Release, 1 Elgin Avenue, London, W9 3DR, for drug education publications.

Pollution and the environment

A minor but not insignificant factor in osteoporosis can be pollution in the environment, affecting your bone mass in two ways: the reduction of sunshine under murky skies (see vitamin D section on p. 96) and the toxic effects of particles of matter in pollution – the aluminium toxicity noted earlier, and especially high levels of lead, cadmium, mercury and zinc. When calcium in the body is low, it tends to be replaced by these other harmful minerals.

Lead. D. Bryce-Smith in *Chemistry in Britain* describes lead as '... one of the most insidiously toxic of the heavy metals to which we are exposed, particularly in its ability to accumulate in the body, and has been said to interfere with practically any life-process one chooses to study.'

When lead enters the bloodstream, about 10 per cent is excreted but the remainder is lodged in bone tissue. Lead can cross the placental barrier to a growing foetus and reach a nursed infant through lactation. It is well-known that high levels of lead in the blood can be fatal, but recent research has found that 30 micrograms per decilitre of blood can have an adverse effect – a level considered free of risk only two years ago. A safe level of lead in the blood has not been established. Unborn children are in danger of acquiring birth defects and children of one to three years of age are most susceptible to permanent damage. It can be absorbed into the body by inhaling, ingesting or through the skin.

Where is lead found? It is in the *air,* mainly from petrol and industrial processes, from burning coal or refuse. Lead is in *food,* from fertilizers, insecticides, pesticides and some ceramic glazes. It may be in *drinking water,* flowing through lead plumbing; and it is in lead-based paints, ammunition, fishing weights and some cosmetics.

What can you do to avoid it? Because children are most at risk from lead pollution, check around the home for old lead-based paint on walls (especially if it is chipping and peeling), or on painted toys, since youngsters tend to chew on paint chips. Unleaded paints are now available in shops for home decorators. In urban areas, lead accumulates in dust, so it is a good idea to do indoor dusting frequently, as well as sweeping porches, steps and driveways where children often play. Be sure that dirty hands are washed before food is prepared, and especially before eating. Buy fresh foods whenever possible, since metallic lead (mainly solder) gets into food during the canning process, particularly if the food is acidic. If you have to use tinned food, wipe the tops of cans carefully before opening; remove food promptly, without scraping the cans too vigorously, and transfer the contents to glass containers. Never store food or juices in tins. All unprocessed fruits and vegetables, from a greengrocer or home-grown, should be thoroughly washed in water or a mild vinegar-water solution, and outer leaves discarded, to remove pesticides, insecticides and contaminated soil as much as possible. If you bake your own pie-shells and pastry-cases using pellets to weight the dough, use glass or ceramic beads or dry beans and not lead or aluminium shot. Discard old toothpaste tubes that sometimes contain lead – more recently, tubes are made of plastic.

If you have lead plumbing, use water only from the cold water tap for the kettle or for food preparation, running it for a few minutes before using. And before installing a water softener, check that you have no lead pipes.

Controversy still surrounds the addition of lead to petrol, to increase the octane rating (in 1986, at the rate of 0.15g per litre), although the practice is a serious health hazard. Australia, New Zealand and the United States now have programmes for marketing lead-free petrol, and it is earnestly hoped that car manufacturers and the petroleum industry will soon reach agreements to ban completely the use of lead additives in the UK, EEC countries and world-wide. Meanwhile leaded petrol continues to be used and to cause concern.

Home potters use lead glazes because other safer glazes require firing at higher temperatures not always achieved with home kilns. If you are buying ceramics at a craft fair, or maybe in a foreign market, ask what kind of glaze was used. Coffee can pull the lead out of lead-glazed coffee mugs, for instance, and poison the person drinking it. Artist-potters may be exposed to glazes that contain the metals lead, cadmium and nickel; they are cautioned to read and follow the directions on labels of art material, use gloves and good ventilation. When glazing vessels intended for food and drink, use a lead glaze on the outside surfaces only, and some other non-toxic glaze on the inside.

Old traditional pewter may have a high lead content and should be avoided for drinking beer, cider or wines, or for storing fruits, pickles and preserves.

Although the sale of lead-containing cosmetics is banned in Britain, leaded eye make-up is still imported from the Indian subcontinent, and some medicines imported from the same area also have a high level of lead.

Cadmium. Cadmium is used in plating steel, iron, copper, brass and other alloys to prevent corrosion. It is used in storage batteries; as pigments in paints, enamels and lacquers. Poisoning can occur after drinking an acidic food or drink, such as lemonade, after preparation in a cadmium-plated can.

In Japan, cadmium poisoning is known as 'Itai-itai' disease, meaning 'it hurts, it hurts'. In the 1960s, cadmium seeped downstream from toxic waste along the Jinzu River, contaminating drinking water and polluting rice paddies near the village of

Haginoshima. When villagers had had repeated pregnancies, severe bone disease developed in old age: calcium from their bones had been drawn off by each growing foetus, and replaced by cadmium, subsequently resulting in bones so weakened that they splinter with a sneeze. The Japanese cadmium dumping ended in 1971, but itai-itai disease is chronic; more than 100 villagers died, and other survivors receive benefits under the Japanese law devised to help people injured by hazardous waste or air pollution.

Closer to home, in Shipham, Somerset, where the village was built over old zinc mines, cadmium concentrations in the soil have been contaminating leafy vegetables and rhubarb. These villagers have now been cautioned to eat less home-grown produce to reduce their intake of cadmium. And in the Heathrow area near London, the use of sewage sludge on market gardens over a long period has increased the cadmium in lettuce and root vegetables. Cadmium is also known to accumulate in kidney meat and in brown crab; other shellfish is being carefully monitored by the Ministry of Agriculture, Fisheries and Food.

Mercury. Even in ancient Egypt mercury was known as a toxic substance, but was used for medical purposes. In the nineteenth century, a mercury compound was used to treat felt in the hat industry, causing poisoning with damage to the kidneys, tremors and other physical effects, hence the term 'mad as a hatter', and subsequently it was banned for that purpose. Today, under carefully controlled conditions, it is used in antiseptic salves, as a germicide, a fungicide, and in diuretics to increase urine flow. Because mercury compounds are presently used in fungicides for seeds, in water-based paints and in paper, the discharge of mercury-containing wastes into drainage systems is creating some concern. Build-up of mercury, through the ecological chain, in tuna, swordfish and salmon, has caused some governments to set definite limits on permissible levels in edible fish.

The Ministry of Agriculture, Fisheries and Food is monitoring the mercury content of fish entering selected British seaports, and reporting to the D.H.S.S.'s Committee on Toxicity.

In the Mediterranean area, high mercury levels previously attributed to industrial wastes, have been found to be originating mainly in natural run-offs from mercury-rich soils, particularly from Spain, Italy, Yugoslavia and Turkey. Under the Mediterranean Action Plan, participating countries have banned dumping of the most dangerous wastes (mercury, DDT, PCBs, arsenic and radioactive substances), but eating raw shellfish in this region is still dangerous.

Zinc. The toxicity of zinc is lower, but still represents a hazard. Zinc is used as a coating for the protection of steel and the production of galvanized metal, frequently seen as a roofing material. It is in tyre production and in weedkillers. Zinc can occasionally enter pipes used for drinking water.

Approximately 63,000 chemical compounds are in common use, with 1000 new compounds added each year to that total. A recent study by the US National Academy of Sciences concluded that 'of tens of thousands of commercially important chemicals, only a few have been subjected to extensive toxicity testing, and most have scarcely been tested at all.' Is there any level of toxicity so low as to be harmless to humans? What is an acceptable risk? Many chemicals can cause cancer, damage to the central nervous system, liver and kidneys, from which it can be inferred that there is an effect on the proper functioning of these organs, impairing bone mineralization.

Write to your government representatives to express your concern; demand an acceleration in efforts to clean up the environment and ensure safe handling and storage of toxic wastes.

Chapter 5

THE CALCIUM CRISIS

Ideally, the way to prevent osteoporosis is to build strong bones before you reach thirty-five, to maintain a strong bone mass through menopause and the later years. The cornerstone of this programme of prevention is CALCIUM, best obtained from the foods you eat. Calcium is needed *throughout* life – vitally important at all ages and for each generation.

What is calcium? The word comes from the Latin 'calx' meaning lime. It is the fifth most abundant element on our planet's crust – never occurring by itself naturally, but always as a compound. Thus as calcium carbonate it occurs in limestone, chalk, marble, dolomite, eggshells, pearls, coral, stalactites and stalagmites, and the shells of many marine creatures. As calcium phosphate, it is the main constituent of bones.

How much calcium do you need?

For the particular needs of the population in Britain, the National Osteoporosis Society recommends the following daily amounts of calcium (Table 4).

Table 4 Daily Calcium Requirements

	Age	*calcium (mg)*
Children	1–12	800
Teenagers	13–19	1200
Pregnant teenagers	13–19	1500
Nursing teenagers	13–19	1500
Women	20–40	1000
Pregnant women	20–40	1200
Nursing women	20–40	1200

	Age	calcium (mg)
Men	20–60	1000
Menopausal women	40–60	(without HRT) 1500
Menopausal women	40–60	* (with HRT) 1000
Men and women	over 60	1200

* Hormone Replacement Therapy: see Chapter 8

These recommendations are meant to represent the amounts of essential nutrients considered adequate for most healthy persons, but they don't take into account *individual* requirements nor the special needs of people who have to follow diets because they are ill or suffering from other medical disorders. Your individual needs of food nutrients depend on many factors – such as your age, sex, size, state of health or disease, and how active you are.

The average woman has a consumption of calcium *far* below the recommended daily intake, with the cumulative effect of giving her a serious calcium deficit.

This is the *Calcium Crisis*!

As you will see later in this chapter, dairy products are the major sources of calcium, but very typically a woman prefers not to eat dairy products as she gets older – either because she mistakenly thinks she has outgrown their need, she considers them too fattening, or perhaps orthodox religion may prohibit their inclusion at certain meals.

At the same time, manufacturers of cola drinks spend millions on powerful advertising promoting soft drinks as part of a youthful, energetic fun-loving lifestyle. But by substituting cola drinks for milk, a woman loses an important source of calcium. For body-conscious women, the smarter choice is milk; milk doesn't have a flashy name and isn't brightly packaged, but it can produce beauty that is more than skin-deep. And for calorie counters, a ¼ pint (150 ml) of regular cola drink is about 59 calories, with only 6mg of calcium, while a ¼ pint of fresh skimmed milk is only 50 calories containing no fat but brimming with 195mg of calcium!

Statistics indicate that the risk of fractures increases with both

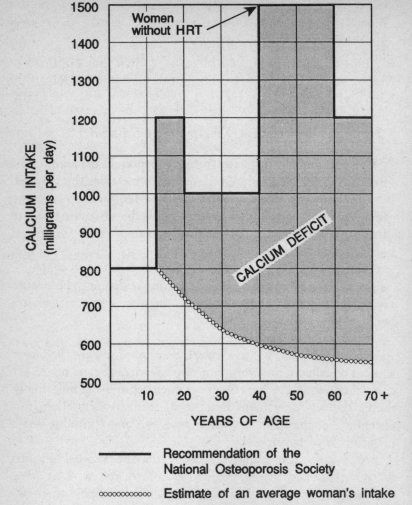

Figure 5

Women and Calcium: The Calcium Crisis

The New Approach to Osteoporosis: A Guide for General Practitioners. (National Osteoporosis Society, 1990).

age and with a reduction of calcium intake. Women who develop porous, pitted, brittle, fragile bones have generally had insufficient calcium, or have had difficulty in absorbing it from their foods.

How much calcium do you absorb?

When you eat food containing calcium, it passes along the gastrointestinal tract, with calcium absorption occurring throughout the length of the small intestine, diffused through the intestinal wall and transported by your bloodstream. The bloodstream carries calcium to body organs and tissues, for vital organ functions, and to storage in the bone cells as mineralization. Calcium is excreted in the urine and stools, and some in perspiration through the sweat glands. How much is actually absorbed by your body to aid mineralization? Absorption of dietary calcium in the intestines is incomplete, ranging from 10 to about 50 per cent of intake, depending on several factors varying with:

- your age, with the differing interplay of hormones,
- your general health and lifestyle, such as habits of smoking and alcohol use,
- your intake of other nutrients such as vitamins,
- your level of emotional stress,
- your level of physical stress and amount of exercise, and
- certain medication you may take for chronic conditions or diseases.

A breast-fed baby receives about 60mg of calcium per kilogram of body weight, and retains 66 per cent of this amount. In contrast, a baby fed formula with standard cow's milk receives about 170mg of calcium per kilogram of body weight, but retains only 25 to 30 per cent. Because of the greater absorption of calcium from human milk, it better fulfils calcium needs.

From the age of one to ten years, the retention of dietary calcium is not as high as during babyhood, but growing children still need about twice as much calcium per unit of body weight as adults do.

Between eleven and eighteen years of age there is usually much accelerated growth of skeleton and muscles, although the retention of calcium can be variable. During these formative years, good nutrition is especially important, with attention paid to daily calcium intake, if the strongest potential skeletal mass is to be attained.

With bone tissue being constantly remodelled, and adult bone not being static, 600 to 700mg of calcium may enter and leave the bones each day.

During pregnancy, in spite of the increased efficiency in absorption, calcium needs are increased above the non-pregnant state. Nutrients, including calcium, are passed to the foetus through the blood circulation of the mother, so it is crucial that a woman has an immediate concern for her extra daily calcium needs as soon as she knows she is pregnant. In fact, it's a good idea to build up calcium levels *before* becoming pregnant. A full-term baby contains about 25 g of calcium: skeletal tissue starts to form during the third month of pregnancy, with most calcium deposited during the last trimester at a rate of 200 to 300 mg daily. Towards the end of pregnancy, when a mother stores additional calcium in preparation for lactation, it is important to continue adequate intake of the mineral.

During breast-feeding, the amount of calcium secreted in breast milk may amount to 250 to 500 mg each day. If a mother has an extremely heavy flow of milk, considerable losses of calcium may occur, making it vital for her calcium to be replenished to safeguard her bones and those of her child.

If you have children in quick succession, with or without breast-feeding, your skeletal mass may be depleted of calcium, especially if you are still adolescent.

Calcium absorption can be influenced by your general level of health, with decreased absorption during an illness and in later years, starting at the age of forty-five for women and sixty in men. Exercise improves calcium absorption, making workouts work better, while prolonged inactivity (such as a long illness) can decrease absorption.

Some medications such as antacids, tetracyclines, laxatives, diuretics, and heparin obstruct calcium absorption.

If you smoke, drink alcohol or many beverages containing caffeine, consume a high-protein diet, use excessive amounts of salt, or have a sedentary lifestyle, you want more calcium, and need extra servings of calcium-rich foods.

During and after menopause, with the changing balance of hormones controlling calcium utilization, coupled with reduced intestinal absorption, and possibly a less active life, calcium requirement is even greater.

Calcium to phosphorus ratio

A good ratio of calcium to phosphorus is about one-to-one. Better yet, would be a calcium-phosphorus relationship of two-to-one, since there is generally an overabundance of phosphorus in today's foods and your body absorbs it more easily than calcium.

Although phosphorus is an essential mineral found in every cell and involved in metabolism, a major component of bone along with calcium, too much phosphorus in excess of calcium intake may lead to a phosphorus-calcium imbalance associated with bone loss. Research with adult animals has clearly shown that too much phosphorus in the diet, or too low consumption of calcium relative to phosphorus, can accelerate bone loss, although this finding in small animals has not yet been established in human beings. Arctic Eskimos of Canada and Alaska lose up to 20 per cent more bone than white Americans, and lose it at an earlier age, where their diet consists largely of walrus and seal meats – rich in phosphorus.

Diet surveys indicate the consumption of two to three times as much phosphorus as calcium, with large intakes of phosphorus derived from meat and animal products, breads and cereals, potatoes, processed foods, beer and soft cola drinks. Many popular foods contain more phosphorus than calcium. Phosphates are in fertilizers, and phosphorus is widely used in food additives and processed foods.

Much phosphorus can be avoided by cutting down (or cutting out) meats and soft drinks, and having fresh whole foods whenever possible. If using processed foods, read nutrition information labels to check the phosphorus content in relation to calcium. Generally, you need to increase your calcium.

Where do you get calcium?

Your body isn't able to manufacture its calcium – you have to obtain it from the food you eat. Absorption of calcium depends largely on the amount you consume and its source. Meats, nuts and grains which contain many other good nutrients, do *not* provide significant amounts of calcium. Best absorption of calcium is from dairy products, but if you eat little dairy food it is still possible to get adequate calcium from green leafy vegetables and other sources, still with an eye to the number of calories involved.

Dairy products

Have at least two servings each day; pregnant and menopausal women, four servings (a serving could be an 8 oz glass of milk, or yogurt, or 1½ oz of cheese).

Check first with your doctor if you take drugs for high blood pressure or depression, as dairy products may not be permitted with some medications such as MAO inhibitors prescribed for depression.

Milk. A ¼ pint (150ml) of skimmed milk will provide about 195mg of calcium. A cup of 'CalciMilk', a lowfat milk fortified with tricalcium phosphate, will have about 300mg. Milk has precisely the right balance of phosphorus and vitamin D to make calcium well absorbed, as well as other nutrients to help your body retain it.

Worldwide, the largest amounts of milk are now produced by the cow and the water buffalo, the latter providing milk in commercial quantities in India. Goats are major milk producers in China, India and Egypt; sheep's milk is used in Southern Europe; reindeer milk is produced in Northern Europe; camels are milked in desert areas, and mares in parts of Asia.

Take advantage of cheap or free milk if you or your family are entitled to it under welfare food schemes. It would be better for most adults to substitute lowfat or skimmed milk, as these products contain all the calcium of whole milk but fewer calories and little of the heart-damaging fats and cholesterol. A few drops of vanilla essence can give it a 'rich' flavour. If you have doorstep delivery, ask your milkman, or in the supermarkets look for labels on cartons that say 'skimmed milk' (less than 0.1 per cent fat), 'semi-skimmed' (less than 2 per cent fat), or 'Vitapint' (to which extra dried milk solids have been added). Paediatricians, however, have given a warning that it is unwise to give young children lowfat or skimmed milk as a general rule, unless upon a doctor's instruction, and fresh milk given before the age of one may cause nutritional problems and allergies.

Be sure to buy *pasteurized* milk to protect you and your family against the harmful bacteria in raw milk. For the most nutrition, don't let milk stay too long on your doorstep; keep it well sealed, refrigerated and away from sources of light.

Ready-prepared chocolate milk is sometimes made from skimmed milk but it can be highly caloric without offering additional calcium. Be wary and read nutrition information labels when buying imitation milk, chocolate drink or chocolate-flavoured drink available in certain areas, as often it is completely synthesized and of little calcium value. Similarly, coffee 'creamers', 'whiteners', or 'lighteners', liquid or powdered, may be of a non-dairy origin, more convenient and possibly cheaper, but without the calcium of a real dairy creamer. If you need speed and convenience without refrigeration, put nonfat dried milk powder in your coffee or tea, as your healthy alternative to fresh milk.

Buttermilk. A cup of buttermilk will provide about the same calcium as a similar amount of standard milk. Originally the milk left over from churning butter, buttermilk is now produced from pasteurized milk to which special bacterial cultures have been added. The bacteria convert part of the lactose (sugar) in milk to lactic acid, resulting in a tart-tasting milk.

Yogurt. 3½ oz (100g) of yogurt will provide about 180 mg of calcium. Yogurt probably originated in the area now known as Turkey. It is made from cow's milk in the UK and North and Central Europe; from sheep and goat's milk in Turkey and South-east Europe; from water buffalo milk in Egypt, from camels in desert areas, and mare's milk in Russia.

The current popularity of yogurt can be said to have originated with a Russian bacteriologist, Ilya Metchnikoff, who was director of the prestigious Louis Pasteur Institute in Paris from 1889 until he died in 1916. Metchnikoff isolated the Bulgarian bacillus in milk that had fermented, in his studies on the remarkable longevity of the Bulgarian people. This bacillus later was named *Lactobacillus bulgaricus.* Yogurt today has to have been cultured by both Lactobacillus bulgaricus and *Streptococcus thermophilus* to be correctly labelled 'yogurt'.

Yogurt is digested in one hour compared to three hours for

milk, because the fermentation of milk into yogurt form partially predigests the milk components.

When calorie-watching, avoid the fruit-flavoured yogurts or those with additional sweeteners; plain lowfat yogurt can acquire flavour interest with the addition of finely chopped fresh fruit, a small spoonful of molasses (or black treacle), or a few drops of vanilla essence to 'suggest' sweetness. To maximize calcium, look for yogurt fortified with nonfat dry milk solids.

Cheese. 2oz (50g) of cheese (Cheddar, for example) will provide about 400mg of calcium. Known for thousands of years before the birth of Christ, the different varieties of cheese are named for the localities where they were first produced. Cheese is a concentrated source of many of the nutrients of milk – a good source of calcium, especially Cheddar. In general, hard cheeses are richer in calcium than the softer varieties. Calorie-watchers can choose the lowfat types such as mozzarella and provolone, while salt-watchers avoid Féta, Parmesan and Romano, and the blue-veined varieties such as Roquefort, Gorgonzola and blue. Heart-conscious readers would be better to use moderation with fatty cheeses.

Ice-cream and ice-milk. Dairy ice-cream can make a delicious contribution to your daily intake of calcium, with 3½oz (100g) providing about 140mg, although the caloric value will vary with the amount of butterfat, cream and sugar in the recipe. Waist-watchers can reduce calories by buying ice-*milk* available in some supermarkets or health-food shops. Read labels, to avoid *non-*dairy ice-cream with little or no calcium content.

Baby food
There is nothing wrong with older people eating certain baby foods for calcium, if you are bored with food or perhaps have problems with ill-fitting dentures. Check the nutrition information labels to make sure of the calcium content needed for an adult.

Green vegetables
Collards, turnip greens, mustard greens, kale, broccoli, all contain a good proportion of calcium, although vegetable sources of the

mineral are not so well absorbed into your system.

It is important to remember that there are some leafy vegetables which would be good calcium sources if it were not for the oxalic acid (oxalates) they also contain, which binds with calcium to block absorption when they are eaten in large amounts. These vegetables include asparagus, beet greens, silverbeet (Swiss chard), dandelion, lambsquarters, parsley, sorrel and spinach – so don't rely on these for calcium. Rhubarb is also in this category of food containing oxalates, reducing calcium absorption.

If you take anticoagulants or thyroid medication, check first with your doctor before eating green leafy vegetables.

Seafood

When eaten with their bones, canned sardines and canned salmon will contribute important amounts of calcium to your diet. Try to select sardines packed in water. If sardines are canned in oil, calorie-watchers and the heart-conscious will drain this off carefully and dress the sardines with vinegar. When using a can of salmon, don't discard the skin and tiny bones as they are all edible and contribute flavour as well as valuable calcium.

Grains and cereals

The calcium content of grain products depends upon which kind of flour is used, the extent to which it has been milled, and whether calcium carbonate has been added. White wheat flour uses mainly the inner kernel while wholewheat flour includes the germ and outer husks. Because the composition of flour in the UK is controlled by certain orders and regulations, calcium carbonate (chalk) must be added to all flours except wholemeal and some self-raising flours, at the rate of about 235–390 mg per 100 g. Many breads and cereals have an enriched calcium content with the addition of nonfat dry milk, so read nutrition information labels, talk with the baker, or write to the food manufacturer.

The outer husks of cereal seeds as in bran contain phytic acid, a substance that forms phytates when combined with phosphorus. Phytates, similar to the oxalates in green vegetables, can interfere with calcium absorption if eaten in excessive quantities. Unlike raw bran, when wholegrain wheat or rye bread is being leavened before baking, the enzyme phytase in the flour splits the phytic acid so that it will not bind with calcium – thereby releasing the calcium to be absorbed and making the bread more nutritious.

Because phytate also occurs naturally in other plant material such as coffee beans and tea leaves, strong infusions of coffee, tea and cocoa have the similar potential to inhibit calcium and zinc absorption, or extract these minerals from your body.

Soya products

Many people say they don't like the taste of milk, or as vegetarians, they don't care to consume food that has an animal origin. Nevertheless your body still has a need for calcium. Get to know the various products made from the soya bean: soya milk, soya flour and especially tofu. (Persons taking thyroid medication should check first with their doctor before eating soya bean products.)

Tofu. 3½oz (100g) will provide about 500mg of calcium. Discovered in China over 2000 years ago, tofu (sometimes called bean curd or bean cake), is the world's most popular soya bean food, serving as a key source of good quality calcium for more than a quarter of the population of the globe, in regions where eating dairy products is not customary. Tofu has only been available in Western health-food stores in the last few years, and more recently in supermarkets. It is easily digested and can safely be eaten by small babies; vegetarians accept it, dieters can reduce calories with it, it is low-sodium and completely free of cholesterol. Serve tofu dishes with wholegrain breads, rice or pasta to complement the protein.

What does it taste like? The taste of tofu changes slightly the longer it is stored. Very fresh, it has a subtle delicate flavour that needs to be well seasoned; older tofu picks up flavours from the other ingredients in your recipes.

Tofu is derived from soya milk curds to which a solidifier has been added, usually gypsum (calcium sulphate) or Epsom salts (magnesium sulphate), similar to the way rennet is added to cow's milk to make cheese. Tofu curds are spooned into moulds to be pressed and cooled. If tofu is not available in the shops in your part of the world, you could produce it yourself if you like gardening, have a space for a patch of soya beans, and the time to devote to tofu making.

Tofu keeps for about a week in its original carton in the refrigerator, but after opening it should be rinsed well, placed in another container, fresh water added and covered. Change the water daily. Tofu can be used to make creamy dips and dressings, as a substitute for all or part of the meat in minced meat recipes, and can substitute for cream cheese, cottage cheese or ricotta. For more information on this calcium-rich food, read *The Magic of Tofu* by Jane O'Brien (Thorsons).

Soya milk. Derived from cooked soya beans pulped in water and sieved, a ¼ pint (150ml) of soya milk has only 8mg of calcium, far below that of cow's milk, but look for calcium-fortified soya milk, preferably unsweetened. It needs refrigeration like cow's milk and has about the same shelf-life, so it can turn sour unless handled with care. Soya milk powder is also available in health-food stores and some supermarkets.

Baby formulas may also be based on soya milk, with good amounts of calcium, easily digestible by all ages (but check with your paediatrician before giving soya milk to a premature baby).

Allergies and lactose intolerance

Allergies

Sometimes so-called 'allergies' are psychological reactions to foods rather than actual physical reactions to real allergies. Milk may be involved in food allergy, although *milk protein allergy* is an uncommon sensitivity generally found in formula-fed newborn babies, which usually disappears at about the age of four. Milk allergy, as with other allergies, *may* develop in later years, but this is rare. Allergic reaction to the *protein* in milk can cause severe diarrhoea, asthma, sneezing or skin rash in susceptible infants after consuming cow's milk. When these symptoms are observed, a paediatrician will immediately change the milk-based formula to one based on predigested protein. Milk products should be entirely eliminated from the diet. Thus label reading is important since milk is often used in convenience foods.

Lactose intolerance

Many people say that 'milk doesn't agree' with them. It's an astonishing fact that, although precise numbers are not available for Britain, at least 30 million Americans are unable to drink milk or consume other dairy products without suffering cramps, bloating and gas. What is the problem? It could be lactose intolerance, pertaining to the natural sugars in milk. The gastric symptoms are very similar for milk protein allergy and for lactose intolerance.

Milk contains a combination of glucose and galactose called milk sugar or *lactose*. (Cow's milk has 4 to 5 per cent; human milk 6 to 7 per cent.) In your intestinal tract are enzymes on the surface of the cell lining that work to digest the different sugars in the diet; and it is the enzyme *lactase* that is necessary to split the sugars in milk, for absorption through the intestinal wall. A shortage of lactase can give many people some difficulty in digesting large quantities of milk and milk products. This is lactose intolerance. If you have insufficient lactase enzymes, and eat large quantities all at one time of foods containing lactose, much of the undigested milk sugar stays in your intestines, with the bacteria present there growing on it and producing gas, similar to the way sugar in wine is fermented by yeast. The result is nausea, stomach ache, cramps, diarrhoea and bloating, that can last up to ten to twelve hours.

Three different types of lactase deficiency are known:

1. *Congenital* lactase deficiency is very rare. In this case, babies are born with limited or no ability to produce lactase, so all lactose-containing foods must be eliminated from the diet.

2. The most common type is caused by a gradual decrease in lactase production after the age of two years, an *inherited* condition which affects millions of people. Members of certain ethnic groups show a definite decline in lactase with age, although lactase production during infancy and early childhood is adequate. But by the time they are teenagers, they have typical symptoms of lactose intolerance. By adulthood, 70 to 75 per cent of blacks, 70 per cent of adult Jews, almost all Orientals and 15 per cent of American Indians and Eskimos are lactase-deficient. Even among Caucasian

populations of Northern European ancestry, lactase deficiency occurs in approximately 5 to 20 per cent of young adults.

Officially, lactose intolerance in the UK has only been noted as a problem for people of African origin, with an estimated incidence of about 1 per cent of the total population. However, according to recent research, most humans have lost much of their ability to make lactase by the time they become young adults, so the problem is clearly shown to be related to ageing. It has been estimated that approximately 80 per cent of the world population is deficient in lactase to some degree. (Consequently it made little sense when the US Government attempted to ship large surplus quantities of dried milk powder to undernourished populations in the Third World, and when the big food corporations producing milk-based baby formulas tried to market their products to poor nations in Africa – a problem compounded by the poor unsanitary sources of water with which to reconstitute the milk and to dilute the formula.)

Many experts believe that lactase deficiency is inherited since some ethnic groups have a high incidence of deficiency while others have a low incidence. Ethnic groups who live in different parts of the world have similar prevalence. For instance, Jews living in the United States have a similar prevalence of lactase deficiency to those living in Israel, and American blacks have a deficiency comparable to that of African blacks.

It is believed that in primitive times, humans seldom drank milk after being weaned. But when some of the world's populations took up dairying, as in Scandinavia and North-western Europe, the people continued drinking milk into adulthood and most of them maintained their capacity to produce lactase. On the other hand, in Southern Europe, Africa and Asia, where milking has been a very recent activity, lactase deficiency is very high, starting as early as the age of three.

The third type of lactase deficiency is not hereditary and may not be permanent, but a temporary condition due to stomach surgery, certain drugs (such as some for arthritis) and antibiotics (particularly penicillin) or radiation treatment in the area of the abdomen. In some cases, where there has been severe damage to the lining of the small intestine, healthy cells are producing lactase but the total produced is insufficient to handle large amounts of lactose. If damaged tissue subsequently recovers to promote growth of healthy lactase-producing cells, lactose tolerance will return to normal.

Your doctor can give you tests in his surgery to check lactose deficiency, or if it is necessary to examine a section of intestinal tissue, an analysis of a small biopsy can be made. But you can do some simple testing for yourself at home.

Early in the day, try drinking two glasses of milk all at once on an empty stomach, and note your system's reactions; with this amount of milk, you will react within an hour or two if you have tolerance. Or cut out all sources of lactose from your diet to see if symptoms disappear, and if they return when consumption of lactose is resumed.

So far, no method has been found to restore general lactase levels. Basic biochemical studies to understand the working of the enzyme lactase have been difficult because it is fragile, but once your problem is identified you will know how to handle it, and very likely you won't have to give up milk and milk products.

If you are sensitive to milk, be sure to check the label of all processed foods for milk, dry milk, buttermilk, cream, casein or dried whey among the ingredients. Be aware that lactose can be found in the following foods, although small portions may often be tolerated.

Drinks:
Milk (whole, lowfat, cream, buttermilk) and yogurt.
Instant coffee, instant cocoa, instant breakfast drinks.
Cream liqueurs and cordials.

Cheeses:
All cheeses, especially lowfat and creamed cottage cheese, gjetost and ricotta.

Meats:
Sausages and luncheon meats containing dry milk.

Liver sausage.
Liver, brain and sweetbreads.
Breaded meat, poultry and fish.
(Kosher meat products and food are milk-free when marked 'pareve')

Fruits and vegetables:
Canned, frozen products in 'cream' sauces, and instant potatoes.

Grain products:
Breads, cereals, crackers, biscuits, pancakes and waffles made with milk.
Prepared mixes for biscuits and scones.

Desserts:
Ice-creams, ice-milk, sherbet made with milk, and milk-based puddings, custards and junkets.
Cakes, pie-crusts, pie-fillings made with milk or cream.

Other:
Cream soups, cream sauces and gravies.
Caramels, chocolates, butterscotch and toffee.
Dietetic and diabetic products.
Milk-based baby foods
Some drug preparations.

Lactose intolerance is *not* like an allergy, where the reaction is unrelated to dose, so you should not have to avoid milk. You need the nutrients of milk, especially its calcium, all your life particularly in later years. The best approach is to determine your own personal level of tolerance to milk, bearing in mind the following:

1. The quantity added to coffee or tea generally gives no trouble. Very often, *small amounts* of milk drunk throughout the day are no problem if taken slowly and in moderation, say ½ cup at a time, and not with other milk products at the meal.

2. If milk is *combined with other foods*, the concentration of lactose is reduced, and the stomach's emptying time is slowed down.

3. If milk is *served at room temperature* or slightly warmed, you will probably tolerate it better than if it is ice-cold. Thus, hot milk is more digestible in cocoa or hot chocolate, cream sauces, cream soups and chowders, puddings and custards.

4. Researchers have now developed *lactose-reduced milk*, cottage cheese and low-lactose milk powder, now available at some dairies, although these products already treated with lactase may not yet be available in many supermarkets.

5. You can treat fresh milk yourself with *lactase enzyme products*: one is called 'LactAid', widely available as drops or tablets, without prescription, from chemists or health-food stores in the UK and around the world. When 'LactAid' is added to milk, after 24 hours the enzyme has broken down 70 per cent of the lactose to make it predigested; after several days, the lactose is reduced by 90 per cent. If added to milk in double the amount specified on the label, the lactose content can be reduced by 95 per cent. This enzyme product will break down lactose in whole milk, lowfat, skimmed, cream, baby formula, goat's milk, condensed and evaporated milk. Enzyme-treated milk can afterwards be used any way you would use ordinary milk, although it does taste sweeter because glucose and galactose (the sugars making up lactose) taste sweeter than lactose. Consequently diabetics should first check with their doctors before using lactase-treated milk products.

6. You can take *milk digestant tablets* containing lactase just prior to eating a lactose-containing food. These tablets are sold in health-food stores or at chemists.

7. Frequently, *fermented milk products* such as buttermilk, sour cream and yogurt are better digested because the fermentation process uses up some of the lactose to grow, producing lactic acid making the characteristic tart taste. This is perhaps why people in other countries who have lactase deficiency usually eat yogurt and other cultured milks. Commercial yogurt has about 60 per cent of the lactose found in the same amount of milk, although there is some variation between brands; in home-made yogurt, you can reduce the lactose content further by prolonging the fermentation period. The advantage

of yogurt is that its healthful bacteria produce the enzyme lactase in the acid-alkaline environment in the stomach, making the nutrients better absorbed.

8. *Cured cheeses* such as natural Cheddar, Gouda and Edam are usually more digestible, because much of the lactose is lost during production. Other low-lactose cheeses are Brie, Camembert, Gruyère, Limburger, Monterey Jack and Port du Salut. Avoid cheeses with the highest lactose content such as lowfat and creamed cottage cheese, gjetost and ricotta.

9. Another way to avoid lactose-containing foods but still consume calcium is to use *soya milk, soya flour* and *tofu*, as detailed earlier.

10. You can obtain your calcium from *supplements* in addition to food.

Calcium without adding pounds (supplements)

'Get your calcium from food from the dairy or grocer and not from the chemist' is the general advice, as your body absorbs dietary calcium more thoroughly than the calcium in supplements. However, for many people that is insufficient for their daily calcium needs. Are you:

- pregnant or breast-feeding your baby?
- convalescent after an illness or surgery?
- on a medically supervised weight-control diet of less than 1000 calories per day?
- a strict vegetarian who avoids all dairy products?
- having dental problems as a result of periodontal disease?
- suffering from a special malabsorption disease?
- over fifty, and finding it difficult to eat sufficient dairy products?

If you answer yes to any of these questions, you should discuss calcium supplements with your physician, to get the vital mineral without consuming more calories. Your doctor can advise you on your personal daily calcium needs, particularly if you are already taking antibiotics or a diuretic, have kidney disease or other intestinal disorders your NHS doctor or clinic may prescribe:

- Calcium lactate gluconate with calcium carbonate (*Sandocal 1000*, 1 tablet daily)
- Calcium carbonate (*Titralac*, 2 to 3 tablets daily)
- Hydroxyapatite (*Ossopan 800*, 4 to 5 tablets daily)
- Calcium carbonate (*Calcichew*, 2 to 3 tablets daily)
- Calcium citrate (*Cacit*, 1 tablet daily)

The amount of calcium in a vitamin–mineral tablet is usually insufficient, since calcium is too bulky to be incorporated in amounts up to 500mg in a vitamin preparation. Supplements come in tablet, powder or liquid form, and are best taken between meals with small amounts of milk or yogurt, which have the lactose and vitamin D to help you absorb the calcium. Since more calcium is lost from your body while you are asleep, be sure to reserve some of the daily supplement for just prior to bedtime — the milk will also help you sleep.

Of the many non-prescription calcium supplements you can buy, most contain one of three calcium compounds (occasionally a combination of them), varying widely in the proportion of calcium they contain. To reduce cost, look for your chemist's own label instead of brand names, and ask the pharmacist for information if the label is insufficient.

Calcium carbonate (40 per cent calcium). This is the highest available concentration of calcium, meaning that generally it is the least expensive because you need to take fewer tablets. This compound is often derived from oyster shells and may contain sweeteners and flavourings. (In Japan, this supplement is often made from tons of pearls, too flawed or tiny for jewellery.) The AMA Division of Drugs recognizes calcium carbonate as the preferred type of oral calcium supplement, although it can cause constipation or gas. Since calcium carbonate needs gastric acid for absorption, the elderly (or those who have had part of their stomachs removed) may find it a problem if their stomachs produce less acid. This compound is commonly used in antacids, and may cause rebound stomach acidity (a vicious circle of acid secretion, antacid, acid, antacid and so on). If you suffer from a chronic duodenal ulcer you may induce excess acid when taking high doses of calcium carbonate.

Calcium lactate (13 per cent calcium). A little more expensive, containing less calcium. Since this compound is usually derived from lactic acid or lactate salts (chemically unrelated to lactose), there should be no problem of lactose intolerance. Calcium lactate appears to be the least gastrically irritating and more soluble for older persons with low stomach acid output.

Calcium gluconate (9 per cent calcium). Because of the small percentage of calcium, it needs to be taken more often throughout the day. It has a very sweet taste.

You will also find in health-food stores or by mail order 'chelated' calcium tablets. Chelation is supposed to improve the absorption in the intestine, anchoring the calcium to other chemicals; it can, however, make the tablets more expensive.

Calcium chloride and calcium levulinate may also be in your health-food store or at the chemist: the first compound can irritate the stomach, and is more used in pickle recipes. The latter, with a low percentage of calcium, has a bitter, salty taste.

Several brands of calcium supplements have the addition of vitamin D to promote calcium absorption. However, D is a fat-soluble vitamin, and it is easy to overdose. Most people acquire sufficient vitamin D through exposure to sunlight, so ask the advice of your doctor on this point. (Read more about vitamin D in chapter 6.)

Bone meal and dolomite These products, usually available as tablets or powder, should be avoided. Bone meal supplements are usually produced from finely milled cattle bone. All bone meal contains a certain amount of lead, originating from the diet of the animal, and generally speaking, there is a greater quantity of lead as the animal gets older. Dolomite is a form of limestone, with a similar risk of lead contamination. The US Food and Drug Administration has issued a warning to doctors and the public about these products connected with the danger of lead poisoning. Since calcium supplements are frequently used by pregnant and nursing women, and by children unable to digest milk, doses of lead can be hazardous, causing effects ranging from anaemia to severe brain damage to death. The lead content in the different brands can be highly variable, according to tests done by the US Consumers

Union in 1982, and dolomite supplements were a little lower in lead than the bone meal products. Although the products are not dangerous by themselves at the recommended dosages, the conclusion was that these particular calcium supplements could add appreciably to the exposure people already have from lead in the air, water and food. If some people exceed the dose, on the principle that more is better, they would have an even higher risk of lead exposure. Even though the prices of bone meal and dolomite are usually somewhat lower than other calcium supplements, the variability of lead in them dictates that they should be avoided, especially as many forms of calcium are available.

How much calcium is too much?

Medical authorities consider that almost everyone can consume 1500mg of calcium daily — but no more than 2000mg — with little risk of adverse health effects, considering an intake *both* from diet and supplements, although no one yet knows the long-term effects of very high supplementation. Symptoms of calcium overdose include constipation, stomach upset, dry mouth, thirst and increased urination. Too much calcium can cause calcification of the arteries (arteriosclerosis) and can create kidney stones if you are predisposed to this problem.

Kidney stones

Although increasing your intake of calcium from foods and supplements is generally considered safe for most people in amounts up to 2000mg per day, consult your doctor before making any radical changes in your diet, as you may be one of the few people prone to forming kidney stones. If you have multiple kidney stones, you have a very real need to cut down calcium intake.

The mechanism of stone formation in adults is a complex phenomenon. Scientists are not always sure why kidney stones form, or why one person has them and another does not, but heredity appears to play an important role in the tendency to form stones. A high level of calcium in the urine often leads to kidney stones. While certain foods may promote stone formation in susceptible people, scientists do not think that eating any specific food causes stones to form in healthy people. Evidence suggests that stones can form because of drinking too little fluid, they may be part of other metabolic disturbances, urinary tract infections, the misuse of certain medications, or lack of exercise of a person subject to stones. Stone formation may also be linked to overactivity of the parathyroid glands or excessive consumption of vitamin D and vitamin C.

According to D.H.S.S. estimates in England in 1983, over 4600 people had hospital treatment for kidney stones; more than a million Americans are hospitalized every year with the problem. Stones seem to occur more often in whites than in black people, in three males for every female; they are also more likely in tropical climates.

What is a kidney stone? Stones, or calculi, may consist entirely of one compound, but most are a combination of various salt or mineral crystals, building up gradually on the lining of the kidneys or urinary tract, possibly causing bleeding of the tissues there and often creating much pain as the stone breaks loose and moves down the urinary tract. When stones grow so large that they cannot be passed out of the body easily, they can obstruct urine, causing acute pain and possible kidney infection or damage.

A doctor's attention is immediately needed to assess the seriousness of the situation. Although in many cases the calculi are passed harmlessly from the body by taking an increased amount of fluids, surgery is often necessary; recent medical advances have increased the possibility that many cases can be cured or controlled with non-surgical techniques such as ultrasonic probes and high-energy shock waves.

Chapter 6

THE VITAMIN SCENE

Calcium absorption is influenced by several constituents in your diet: phosphorus, fat, protein, lactose, fibre, fluoride, magnesium – and most significantly, vitamin D. Vitamins A and C also are important in bone formation, but their relationship to osteoporosis is less clearly established.

If you are pregnant, nursing, or have young children, take advantage of the vitamin tablets or drops (which usually contain vitamins D, A and C) available free or at a reduced price at your local Child Health Clinic or Welfare Food Distribution Centre.

Vitamin D

Vitamin D is vital for the absorption of calcium into your body for proper bone mineralization. The D.H.S.S. has no recommendation for adult intake of vitamin D, but children, adolescents, pregnant/lactating women and the housebound need 10 micrograms daily.

You get most of your vitamin D from the *sun*, with the ultraviolet (UV) light in sunshine converting a substance in your skin to a pre-vitamin D. This pre-vitamin is then changed in the liver and kidneys to its active form, the hormone calcitriol, necessary to maintain constant blood calcium levels for the normal functioning of nerves and muscles. Your body is not actually synthesizing vitamin D while you are in the sunshine, as it takes three or four days for your system to complete the process and 'recharge your batteries'. How much sunshine are *you* getting every day?

Invisible UV light cannot penetrate ordinary window glass, so in order to soak up those rays you have to be outdoors. The Earth's surface is protected by the upper layers of the atmosphere with ozone molecules in the stratosphere absorbing most of the near ultraviolet. Pollution at ground level may increase the ozone layer still further and interfere with the overall strength of the radiated light, so it is difficult to measure how much UV you are getting.

According to a research team at Harvard Medical School, you need about fifteen minutes to one hour of sun exposure each day, to fill your vitamin D needs, if you are a lightly pigmented person. Transmission of light depends on the thickness of your skin's outer layers. After you reach the age of forty or fifty, there is a steady decline in the ability of your skin to produce that pre-vitamin D, as your skin thins with age (coupled perhaps with a lesser performance from your liver). So the skin of a woman in her seventies makes about half the vitamin D produced by her twenty-year-old granddaughter under the same conditions.

There are many variables: How intense is the sun? Is it winter or summer? Do you live in a northern latitude or the 'Sun Belt'? The incidence of hip fracture is highest in the north of Scotland and lowest in the south of England, in studies related to the hours of sunshine and its effect on body stores of vitamin D.

Are you at a high altitude? At high altitudes and near the equator, the UV level is greater than at sea level or in northern latitudes. How clear is the air? Do you have smog and pollution? The low angle of a winter sun blocks much of that UV light, as the rays have to pass through more of our planet's ozone layer, and smog, smoke and fog can block out still more UV.

Do you have a light or a dark skin? If your skin is naturally dark with the pigment melanin, it can screen off as much as 95 per cent of the UV light from the skin layers making pre-vitamin D. It is estimated that a black person needs five times as much exposure to the sun as a fair-skinned person to produce the same amount of vitamin D. When darker pigmented people move from the south to the lower intensity of a northern sun, they can become vitamin D-deficient. For instance, Arab and Indian women, accustomed to living in seclusion or heavily veiled, have been found deficient in the vitamin when going to live under the cloudy skies of Britain. So let the sun get to your bones!

As the sun is at its strongest and most harmful between 10 a.m. and 2 p.m., sunning in the early morning or late afternoon is less damaging to your skin than the middle of the day.

If you use one of the sunblockers or sunscreens, wait about fifteen minutes when out in the sun before applying. These preparations may prevent the sun-related production of vitamin D in your skin.

Beware of excessive sunbathing which is both unnecessary and unhealthy. Most people think it fashionable and fun to be tanned. Millions of fair-skinned people now live in the 'Sun Belt' though their skin may be sun-sensitive and burn rapidly.

Sunlamps and sunbeds using UV light have been popular for providing a tan in winter and more recently tanning salons have been established in some cities. Dermatologists agree that concentrated doses of UV can cause skin damage, so the potential for short- or long-term injury is there, whether the UV radiation is from sun or lamp, with the result being premature wrinkles and, more seriously, a risk of malignant melanoma. This once-rare cancer has been doubling about every twelve years since World War II with a death rate in women faster than from any other malignancy other than lung cancer. Queensland, Australia, had an influx of fair-skinned people after World War II, and seven to ten years later they saw a large increase in melanoma there. If you notice any changes in colour or size of moles or scar tissue, see your doctor immediately.

The elderly need to take special precautions against overexposure to the sun and high temperatures, particularly if you are obese or have diabetes or heart disease. Certain types of drugs can create a vitamin D deficiency, but others when combined with excessive sunshine, can bring on photosensitive or phototoxic effects. Drugs that can create problems when taken along with heavy doses of sunshine are: some tranquillizers, anti-hypertensives, diuretics, tetracycline antibiotics, sulpha drugs, oral diabetic drugs and quinidine. If you are taking any prescription or non-prescription medicines, check first with your doctor or pharmacist for possible reactions in strong sunlight.

And make sure your eyes are protected during sunning – research suggests that prolonged exposure to UV over many years can contribute to the premature development of cataracts and tumours.

Getting a healthy exposure to sunshine every day is the best way for your body to acquire vitamin D, but there are dietary sources if you can't get outdoors or if skies are smoggy.

Because medical authorities were concerned several years ago about possible deficiencies in vitamin D, with few natural sources in food, it was decided to fortify certain items. Margarines and lowfat spreads are required by law to be fortified with 2.25 micrograms of vitamin D per ounce. Some dairies and food firms also fortify skimmed or semi-skimmed milk, evaporated milks, yogurts, dried milk powders and breakfast cereals.

Other foods with naturally present vitamin D are some saltwater fish (herrings, salmon and sardines, for instance), cod-liver oil and halibut-liver oil, egg yolks, liver and cheese.

Vitamin D is stable in cooking and not lost by heating or processing, but it is affected by rancidity in oils. Hence if oils, butter and margarine become rancid, the active vitamin is destroyed.

For better absorption, it's more desirable to get this vitamin from sunshine, but you may need supplementary amounts of vitamin D, especially in winter, if you are:

● breast-feeding, or
● elderly, living in a town or housebound,
● a shift-worker (nurse, for example) working mainly at night,
● heavily wrapped in clothes,
● rarely eat dairy products,
● using heavy make-up.

The NACNE report (from the National Advisory Committee on Nutrition Education) also recommends that Asian schoolchildren be given vitamin D supplements.

By springtime you may have depleted your store of vitamin D. Records indicate that bones fracture most frequently in winter and early spring, when daylight is short, sunshine scarce and when vitamin D and calcium reserves are low. Multi-vitamin preparations usually contain vitamin D, and calcium supplements are often augmented by the vitamin.

However, you can have too much of a good thing: because vitamin D is fat-soluble and stored in the liver, large quantities from over-supplementation can be toxic, cause kidney damage, or trigger the creation of kidney stones. The toxic dose varies among individuals, but toxicity has occured at levels as low as 50 to 125 micrograms daily. When large amounts of vitamin D supplements (over 25 micrograms) are taken without sufficient calcium, bone depletion may occur. (In contrast, your skin has a built-in system that shuts down synthesis of vitamin D after a certain amount of UV exposure, eliminating the danger of toxic effects from sunning.)

Discuss your needs with your doctor before embarking on any tablet supplementation.

Vitamin A

This vitamin is responsible for your vision in dim light, helping you to see in the dark, but it is also needed to make bones grow properly to their correct length. How much do you need? The D.H.S.S. has established the Recommended Daily Amount for adults at 750 micrograms (retinol equivalent); a woman needs 1200 micrograms while breast-feeding. Unless you are a nursing mother, amounts over 1000 micrograms a day may trigger bone loss.

Vitamin A must by law be added to margarines and lowfat spreads in the amount of 255 micrograms per ounce. Vitamin A may also be in skimmed milks, dried milk powder and yogurts to offset the loss of the vitamin when milkfat is removed.

Vitamin A is also found in liver (beef, chicken and lamb) and liver sausage, yellow fruits (such as apricots, cantaloupe melons, mangoes, nectarines, papayas and peaches) and yellow vegetables (such as carrots, pumpkin, sweet potatoes, winter squashes and yellow varieties of sweet corn).

Because it is fat-soluble and stored in the liver and fat cells of your body, it is important not to overdose on this vitamin. Prolonged excessive intake may trigger bone loss, as well as cause diarrhoea, liver damage, drowsiness, headaches, loss of hair and nausea. Avoid eating large quantities of liver, yellow fruits and yellow vegetables – especially during summer when produce is plentiful.

Liver is particularly high in vitamin A. An example of that is the story of some starving Arctic explorers who ate the livers of dogs which had been fed whale meat, and were poisoned by the concentration of vitamin A stored in the dogs' livers. Such an incident is unlikely to recur, however, as foods in the UK do not contain such toxic amounts of vitamin A. Nevertheless, large amounts of vitamin A are particularly dangerous, and to be avoided for good bone health.

The vitamin A content in foods is not reduced by normal cooking; quickly steamed vegetables will have the maximum, but frying in oil will cause some loss. Canning and freezing have little effect on vitamin A content, but sunshine causes destruction, with sun-dried foods having a much reduced amount of the vitamin compared with commercially dried fruits.

Vitamin C
You need plenty of foods rich in this vitamin, also known as ascorbic acid. Vitamin C is utilized by your body for the production of collagen forming connective tissue; this vitamin will help if you have bone fracturing, sore or bleeding gums, or wounds that fail to heal. When our bodies evolved, they were not designed to store vitamin C for any length of time (because fruits and vegetables were plentiful), so the body needs vitamin C daily. The adrenal gland has a high level of vitamin C, and it is known that, in stressful situations, as the production of hormones goes up in this gland, its level of vitamin C goes down. Oral contraceptives, or overuse of laxatives, can decrease your absorption of vitamin C, with consequent reduced levels of this vitamin. Osteoporosis can develop from such nutritional disorders as scurvy, vitamin C deficiency; although only a few elderly people develop scurvy, many more have low reserves of this vitamin.

How much vitamin C do you need each day? The recommendation of the D.H.S.S. for adults is 30 mg, with 60 mg for pregnant women and nursing mothers.

There are between 50–60 mg of vitamin C in ½ cup of orange juice or one medium orange. Orange-flavoured breakfast drinks can be misleading, with many advertised as having more vitamin C than orange juice, but they have little else but vitamin C and sugar, with more calories. And the 'juice' in which fruit is canned, usually a sugar-water syrup, has no vitamin value. Real unsweetened orange juice has vitamin C plus other natural minerals and nutrients, so check the labels.

Other produce with this vitamin are: citrus fruits and natural citrus juices, blackcurrants, kiwifruit, canned pineapple juice and cranberry juice cocktail (but little in prune juice). Potatoes, especially baked and eaten with the skin, contribute substantial amounts of vitamin C. Other good sources are fresh picked tomatoes, tomato juice, green peppers and fresh green leafy vegetables.

Since water-soluble vitamin C is easily destroyed by heating, fruits and vegetables not eaten raw should be lightly cooked or steamed for a short time only. Carefully refrigerate leafy vegetables and don't leave them soaking in water before cooking. Generally, more vitamin C is retained if cooking is in a microwave oven, well covered, than on a conventional stove-top.

Canned fruits and vegetables have generally lost some of their vitamin C through processing; some brands may have extra ascorbic acid added to make up the losses. Check the labels. Frozen fruits and vegetables will usually retain good amounts of vitamin C during freezing – but drying to preserve foods will destroy this delicate vitamin.

Small amounts of vitamin C are naturally present in milk, but 25 per cent is destroyed by pasteurization, with further losses in the heat process for UHT milk and sterilization. Don't leave bottled milk on the doorstep in sunlight – substantial amounts of vitamin C can be lost. Don't rely on milk alone to supply you with this vitamin.

It has been several years since Dr Linus Pauling wrote his book *Vitamin C and the Common Cold* advocating megadoses of vitamin C. Many subsequent studies, however, have shown no benefits from this practice. In fact, taking more than 1 gram daily can result in acidic urine and encourage the growth of kidney stones. Some studies show that high dosage vitamin C can change the level of oestrogen in oral contraceptives, according to Dr Daphne A. Roe, Professor of Nutrition at Cornell University, USA.

Chapter 7

THE VALUE OF EXERCISE

Now let's turn to the big E that stands for EXERCISE, very necessary in maintaining a positive calcium balance.

During the past 100 years, machines have taken over most of the work previously done by human muscles. Labour-saving devices have taken on the manual labour in factory and home. Cars and buses have eliminated walking and bicycling. Lifts and escalators make stair climbing unnecessary. Fewer and fewer people have the hard labour of farm work; many sit to get to work, sit at an office all day, sit for meals, then sit in front of a TV or cinema screen.

But the body was designed to *move*, and physical activity is necessary to preserve bone mass.

A sedentary life can ruin your health, increasing the likelihood of muscle and bone deterioration, heart disease, obesity and premature ageing. Prolonged minimal physical activity can produce a calcium deficit, with losses of calcium mostly from weight-bearing bones. Excessive pounds can put an added burden on already weakened bones.

The good news is that it is almost never too late to do something about it. Regardless of age, studies show that exercise can help you, even if you are bed-ridden, confined to a wheelchair or somewhat handicapped. Tissues of all ages respond to resumed stimulus with vigour and renewal, as muscle is strengthened and bone density increases.

Young people should get plenty of exercise while their skeletal mass is still reaching maturity; adults need to continue exercise to maintain and strengthen their musculature and bone mass; and exercise is particularly important to older women who may be susceptible to osteoporosis and fracturing of bones. A common type of low back pain has been traced to weakened back muscles; exercise can bring relief and help prevent occurrences.

Exercise delays the loss of muscle tissue which in turn slows the demineralization of your bone mass, even to increasing the density of bones. It should come as no surprise that studies of athletes show they have greater musculature and denser bones than people leading a sedentary life. It has been suggested that the need for exercise actually increases with age, because as body processes and systems become less effective over the years, exercise should make up this reduction in efficiency by stimulating metabolism. But most people's level of physical activity seems to decrease, and it is easy to find an excuse for sitting in an armchair. Many people have exercise deficiency and are unaware of it.

Exercise can:

- accelerate the flow of blood to your bones, to transport nutrients for bone building and increasing new bone growth,
- strengthen and tone your muscles, so that everything you do will seem easier,
- help reduce blood pressure,
- act as a transquillizer releasing tension, reducing stress and lowering the production of harmful adrenal hormones,
- help you sleep better, without using pills,
- help you ward off depression, and give a sense of well-being; you'll *feel* better because you'll be healthier, and know you're looking better, with glowing skin and more upright posture,
- help decrease body fat and re-shape your body. More significant than the numbers on your bathroom scales will be the change in the composition of your body tissue as you go from fat to fit.

If you've been sedentary for an extended period of time, first get approval from your doctor before starting any exercise programme. Your physician is in the best position to suggest the type of activity best for you, its intensity and duration, beginning at an easy level. A vigorous workout for someone else could be hazardous for you; overexercising is dangerous and impractical. Jogging, for instance, would not be suitable if you have a history of heart disease or if you are already osteoporotic, since the activity could severely jar your frame. Check also with your doctor if you are already athletic and want to step up your training programme, since too vigorous activity could unbalance your hormone production, with loss of oestrogen and menstrual periods, triggering loss of bone calcium reserves.

Exercise and movement doesn't have to be rapid or difficult to be effective – even house cleaning can help by bending and stretching your body to *move* it. For maintaining healthy bones, choose an activity that calls for pull and stress on the long bones of your body: aerobics, bicycling, skipping and walking.

Exercising should be fun and enjoyable, doing the things that *you* want to do in your spare time, making it part of your lifestyle and not a special short-lived programme. Exercise should be on a steady daily basis, or at least three or four times a week, not a surge of effort just at weekends.

Do you prefer an outdoor or an indoor activity? And what time of day suits you? Taking into account your own biological clock, the best time to exercise is either early morning or late afternoon, avoiding midday heat or late-night exertions that may keep you awake. Always pay attention to what your body tells you. If you feel uncomfortable, you are probably trying to do too much. Take a break and resume at another time or another day. Try different activities and times before deciding on your fitness routine and making it part of your day. A variety of exercise will keep you interested, not bored, so you stay the course.

Do you want to join an exercise group, exercise with a friend, or exercise alone with TV or video tape? If you exercise alone, and you are elderly, tell someone in case you need assistance. Joining a group can make exercise more fun and stimulating; there are many different organizations offering classes. Ask your local authorities what sports are available at nearby centres:

- church or synagogue,
- civic centre, recreation centre or senior citizens' centre,
- local college or Further Education authority,

- YMCAs and YWCAs,
- your firm's recreation club,
- private clubs.

Before joining, attend a class to watch. Is the instructor about your age? Are the people in the class about your age and level of fitness? What are the objectives of the group? What do they think of the programme of exercise? When you do join, don't compete with others, as each of you is responding to exercise in a different way. Only compete with yourself to bolster your improvements. For aerobics, never dance with bare feet. Avoid injury by wearing correct shoes to cushion the balls of your feet and make sure the floor is carpeted over padding.

If you think that regular exercise classes are not for you, there are other ways to stay fit: walking and hiking; bicycling, outdoors and inside on an exercycle; dancing, jazz and square dancing; tennis and squash; and exercise with machines such as Nautilus equipment.

Walking, as briskly as possible, is perhaps the most convenient and beneficial exercise if you are older – almost everyone can do it, almost anywhere, almost anytime, and it doesn't cost anything. It places little strain on your heart and joints while improving the functioning of your muscles and bones, and benefiting your cardiovascular system. Get yourself some good walking shoes – with sturdy heels, flexible rubber soles, and uppers made of materials that 'breathe' such as leather or nylon mesh. Walk wherever it is the most pleasant and convenient in your neighbourhood, but preferably not city streets that would expose you to too much air pollution from vehicles and dust.

Think about the amount of walking you actually do each day and how small changes in your habits can increase the activity: leave the car in the garage, and walk to the shops, to the railway station or to work. Walk the dog. Walk to visit a neighbour. Walk to the newsagent for the daily newspaper instead of having home-delivery. If you take the car for shopping, park in the furthest slot and not the closest to the supermarket. Park half a mile from your office building and walk the remainder; then increase the distance from work as your energy increases. At your work place, walk up stairs instead of taking the lift, and in your lunch break, instead of talking get walking!

If weather is bad and you have to stay indoors, there's no need to abandon exercise. Have a *treadmill* for long-distance walking, right in your living room or office. Some models change angles so that as well as level walking you can give yourself the extra challenge of going uphill or downhill.

Exercise bicycles and *rowing machines* are often better than hard-impact exercise if you have joint or foot problems. Exercise bicycles can take up little space in the corner of a room, and some fold away smaller still, fitting into the tiniest of cupboards. (However, *don't* store your equipment – you may forget to use it!) Some have magazine racks for reading while cycling, to stave off boredom, and movable hand-levers to work upper arms as well as legs. There are bicycles that not only measure speed and distance, but also tell you the time spent cycling, calories expended, pulse rate and work rate (calories per hour).

Weight-training can be with elaborate machines, with heavy weights tied to wrists or ankles, or with simple devices such as a couple of soup cans.

Swimming can be a gentle way of embarking on an exercise programme and is beneficial if you are already osteoporotic or arthritic, for flexing your muscles, and helping stiff joints, while being buoyed by the water. Build up gradually with short swim sessions until you can be more vigorous.

Whatever activity you do, be sure to have warm-up and cool-down periods, so that muscles are limbered up and not strained, and the pace of your heart and lungs speeds up and then returns to normal. Regular stretching can be for everyone, to prevent muscle strain or injury, improving circulation and increasing your range of motion, while relaxing you.

Your body contains 200 bones and 600 different muscles, all benefiting from exercise to some extent. Medical opinion is agreed that most of us should be more active, and it's never too late to start. You don't have to buy fancy home equipment or join expensive clubs to be fit. Whatever you do will bring dividends. While running and aerobics may be too strenuous if you are elderly, make small changes in your lifestyle to put more activity into your day.

If you are already doing some form of exercise, how does it

rate for its contribution to strengthening your muscles and bones and giving you flexibility?

For more on exercise, read *Weight Training for Women* and *Weight Training for Men*, both by Tony Lycholat (Thorsons).

Chapter 8

HORMONE REPLACEMENT AND OTHER THERAPY

While research continues on osteoporosis, it is not possible to say whether it is due solely to calcium malnutrition, lack of exercise or hormone deficiency, but probably it will be found to be an interplay of all three factors. Each woman is unique with her individual needs and concerns.

There has been a great deal of confusion and controversy concerning hormone therapy to prevent osteoporosis, with research still being carried out and new aspects continually being discovered.

The term 'Oestrogen Replacement Therapy' was formerly used, but since it was realized that therapy frequently involves more than oestrogen, the terminology 'Hormone Replacement Therapy' (HRT) is preferred by physicians.

If you are at high risk of developing brittle bones in later years, with many of the negative factors that cannot be eliminated, when calcium absorption may be insufficient and exercise impossible, discuss hormone replacement therapy with your physician. HRT is available under the National Health Service, and may be prescribed by your GP or NHS clinic. Your doctor will probably strongly recommend hormone replacement therapy if:

- your menstrual periods stopped at an early age; or
- you have had surgery to remove your ovaries, effecting a surgical menopause; or
- you have had bone-mass tests at regular intervals that reveal an increasing porosity and risk of fracturing.

Just what is HRT, what are the good points and what are the

bad? Chapter 2 describes the 'balance sheet' of hormones for bone formation, with oestrogen and progesterone from the ovaries on the positive side. It's natural for ovaries to start producing hormones at puberty and wind down production at menopause. It's a misconception that you produce no more natural oestrogen and need full replacement of this hormone at that time. In many menopausal women, ovaries still produce oestrogen, but in insufficient amounts to menstruate. When your ovaries stop making oestrogen, you are not completely lacking this hormone from other sources in your body. Oestrogens come

(a) from the adrenal cortex in the adrenal gland (precursors of oestrogens);

(b) indirectly from the body's fat cells which convert androgens to oestrogens; and

(c) from your ovaries (unless you have had them surgically removed), continuing to manufacture small quantities of androgens which are converted to oestrogens.

While it is true that the quantity of oestrogen drops, the big questions are whether this deficiency needs to be replaced, and if such replacement is safe.

It is important to ask probing questions of your physician if hormone replacement therapy is suggested, so you are aware of all the facts to make an informed decision. Know both sides of the issue and get a second opinion from another physician before reaching any conclusions. A decision made now may need re-evaluating years hence if you experience severe deterioration in bone mass or if particular drugs are later produced that may be suitable for you.

Hormones for retarding bone loss

It is now the commonly shared view of many experts that oestrogen hormones are highly effective for the prevention of osteoporosis, reducing bone resorption and retarding post-menopausal bone loss. Doctors are finding 60 per cent fewer fractures of the hip and wrist among older women who started low-dose oestrogen therapy within a few years of menopause. Studies also suggest that oestrogen reduces the rate of vertebral fractures. Even when therapy is begun six years after menopause, oestrogen stems further decrease of bone mass – although it does not restore it to pre-menopausal levels. But there is no convincing evidence yet that osteoporosis will be prevented if oestrogen therapy is started in very elderly women.

Replacement oestrogen can give relief of hot flashes, drenching perspiration, vaginal dryness, and have a major protective effect against cardiovascular disease in postmenopausal women — an important consideration in this age group.

How do you take hormones?

Discuss fully with your physician the different ways of using hormones. Oestrogens are most often in tablet form and taken by mouth. They may be from natural sources or artificially produced synthetics. Hormones can also be injected or implanted beneath your skin, or placed under the tongue (sublingual) or applied as a dermal patch (sticking plaster) to non-hairy skin or near the buttocks, allowing the drug to be absorbed through the skin directly into the bloodstream at a constant rate. When oestrogen is taken on its own, doctors refer to it as 'unopposed', and current opinion is that it should be balanced by taking progestin (the synthetic form of progesterone) a few days each month to mimic the normal premenopausal ovarian cycle. Progestin now plays an important part in a hormone replacement programme. With this system, some of the risks of side effects are lessened, but the drawback is that you may menstruate every month. Drug manufacturers are now producing 'conjugated' oestrogens with a balanced formula.

Ask your doctor if your treatment would be for a short term only, or whether long-term therapy is being considered, what the minimum dosage would be, and whether your risk of bone loss is sufficiently high that it outweighs the risk of side effects. The best evidence suggests that 0.625mg of conjugated oestrogen daily (not the mega-doses once prescribed) in addition to adequate dietary calcium, is necessary to maintain skeletal mass in white women. Your doctor can adjust the prescription to suit your personal needs. Since studies on dosage have been based almost entirely on white women, treatment of women from other racial backgrounds is best determined on an individual basis.

What are the risks associated with hormone therapy?

While there seems to be little doubt that hormone therapy can be beneficial in the treatment of osteoporosis in postmenopausal women, there are significant hazards that have to be considered. Oestrogen is a powerful chemical which has an impact on many systems in the body.

If you have had serious problems in the past with oral contraceptives, then oestrogen or hormone therapy should perhaps not be undertaken. Hormone therapy probably would not be prescribed if you are overweight, have high blood pressure, varicose veins, seizure disorders, diabetes, liver or gallbladder disease, undiagnosed vaginal bleeding, migraine headaches, or smoke heavily.

There is an increased risk of *blood clotting*. Since oestrogens are usually taken orally, they go immediately to the liver in a relatively high concentration, overstimulating this organ.

Oestrogens used in menopausal therapy and high-oestrogen birth-control Pills have both been linked to *cancer of the endometrium*. During the years you are menstruating, one of the normal effects of natural oestrogen is stimulation of the lining of the uterus (endometrium), and in the menstrual cycle progesterone is produced as a counterbalance, triggering the shedding of the uterus lining. When the stimulation caused by oestrogen supplements is 'unopposed' by progestin, it can produce an overgrowth or thickening of the endometrium which can precede endometrial cancer, especially if you have never borne a child. This risk can be diminished, however, if oestrogen therapy is supplemented with progestin. If you have a family history of endometrial cancer, or if you are overweight (and producing oestrogens derived from your androgen hormones), or if you have a menstrual cycle that does not naturally produce progesterone, you would be at high risk when taking unopposed oestrogens.

If, on the other hand, your family has a medical history of heart disease, women's natural hormones apparently give protection before menopause; but when hormone production stops, the rate of women's heart disease quickly rises to equal that of men. And while oestrogen supplements appear to reduce heart disease risks, combined oestrogen/progestin therapy can erase the cardiovascular protection of oestrogen.

Another side effect may be tender swollen breasts and the possibility of *breast cancer* after long-term therapy (although this is controversial among medical researchers). If other female members of your family have had breast cancer, or if you have a tendency to have cystic breasts, you may have an increased danger of developing cancer of the breast if prescribed oestrogens. A Swedish study reported in 1989 showed that women taking a combination of oestrogen/progestin for more than six years were more than four times as likely as other women to develop breast cancer.

If you take hormones for more than a year, you may have a deficiency of vitamin B_6, which can give you a feeling of *depression*. This deficiency can be offset by eating organ meats, wholegrain breads and dark leafy vegetables, or taking a folate supplement.

Other drawbacks to hormone therapy can be weight increase, fluid retention and headaches, but a low-sodium diet can help in many cases. Your doctor may also mention other side effects of nausea, vomiting, abdominal cramps and dizziness.

Before starting hormone therapy, your physician will give you a thorough examination including tests for liver disease, hypertension or heart disease, existing breast or endometrial cancer that would rule out the taking of oestrogen supplements. There should be a Pap test of your cervix and a suction curettage of your uterus, with a biopsy to ensure there are no cancerous or precancerous cell tissues or pre-existing fibroids.

During therapy you will need to be under close surveillance by your physician, with examinations every six months. Mammography, Gravely jet-washing of the uterus or further biopsies may be necessary to ensure there is no development of cancer and for tests to evaluate your rate of bone loss. If undesirable thickening of the endometrium occurs, your doctor can reduce dosage or change the type of hormone. Any unusual blood spotting should immediately be reported to your physician. If therapy is begun while you are still menstruating, your usual bleeding pattern should continue, and may extend into your sixties.

Summary

If you decide on hormone replacement therapy, try to have the smallest possible dosage for the shortest possible time to avoid the possibility of cancer – but sufficient to maintain bone mass. The preferred method to minimize risks is to have natural oestrogens in conjunction with progestin on a monthly cycle, but there is as yet little information about the safety of long-term treatment.

With hormone treatment containing risks, it should not be considered routine for all women, but if you are at high risk of developing brittle bones, there is no doubt that it can be extremely valuable.

In April 1984, a US Government-sponsored Conference on Osteoporosis attended by eminent research specialists and physicians, issued a consensus statement: 'Until more data on risks and benefits are available, physicians and patients may prefer to reserve oestrogen (with or without progestogen) therapy for conditions that confer a high risk of osteoporosis, such as the occurrence of premature menopause.'

If you decide not to have HRT, make sure you have dietary calcium up to 1500mg daily, with adequate vitamins D and C, and plenty of exercise to keep bones strong. If you are prescribed HRT, your doctor may consider that 1000mg of calcium, plus vitamins and exercise, is sufficient.

Other therapy for osteoporosis

Fluoride. The study of sodium fluoride in therapeutic doses (in association with a high calcium intake) for the treatment of osteoporosis is still in an experimental stage and has not been established as standard practice, nor precise dosage determined. According to current reports, it accelerates new bone formation in patients with osteoporosis, when used in combination with calcium and vitamin D. However, not all patients respond to this therapy, the new bone tissue apparently tends to break easily, and patients report side effects of rheumatic joint pains, vomiting and nausea sufficiently troublesome to abandon the fluoride treatment.

Calcitonin. Injections of synthetic calcitonin have been given experimentally to osteoporotic women but the treatment has been found ineffective after about one year as resistance to its beneficial effects was built up. Skin allergies have been reported, and the high cost of the drug limits its usefulness. A nasal spray is being developed.

Calcitriol (vitamin D). Because large amounts of vitamin D relative to calcium intake may stimulate an increase in bone demineralization, or stimulate the formation of kidney stones, activated vitamin D may only be prescribed by a doctor thoroughly familiar with this method.

Androgens (or anabolic steroids). Recent studies indicate they might be helpful in slowing the rate of bone loss; however, the US Food and Drug Administration has withdrawn approval for their use in treating osteoporosis. Oral preparations may cause liver problems. Although the results of long-term usage of this therapy are not available, patients have observed side effects such as additional growth of hair on face and body, signs of acne and voice-deepening. These effects can be minimized by taking the drug for three weeks, then discontinuing for one week.

Magnesium. Research using magnesium for increasing calcium absorption has had contradictory results.

Testosterone enanthate. Osteoporosis in men can be treated by your doctor with this hormone, although it may create symptoms of prostate cancer.

Etidronate. Still undergoing clinical trials in several countries, the drug etidronate appears to coat bone surfaces, inhibiting the normal process by which the body dissolves and resorbs bone into the bloodstream.

Research continues . . .

A major goal of research is to learn enough about the causes of osteoporosis so that women who have indications of it can be identified and treated promptly. Researchers hope to gain a profile of women at highest risk of fracturing to pinpoint those for whom preventive therapy would be most beneficial. Programmes have a two-pronged thrust:

1. to identify those with greatest risk so preventive steps can be taken, and

2.   prompt treatment after diagnosis, before bone loss becomes irreversible.

Bone growth and remodelling will be studied, and it is hoped to develop safe, effective, low-cost means to maximize peak bone mass, minimize bone loss, and prevent fractures.

Genetic-engineering companies are researching proteins to help the body's natural bone-repair mechanisms, or producing other proteins called BMPs (bone morphogenetic proteins), designed actually to promote growth of new bone cells, to strengthen bones that have become less dense and brittle.

Chapter 9

WHEN YOU KNOW YOU HAVE BRITTLE BONES

You may have already suffered some deformity from brittle or porous bones, have lost some height and be stooped. Unfortunately, there is no way to repair crushed vertebrae, expand a spine already compressed, or straighten a 'dowager's hump' (although researchers are experimenting at the University of North Carolina, Chapel Hill, with a new 'artificial bone' that is a blend of plaster of Paris and fired ceramic particles of hydroxyapatite, the primary calcium compound in bone).

Repairs of hip fractures can be made: broken sections of bone can be pinned or screwed, and severe fractures may dictate that part of the femur (thigh bone) be replaced. Having had an osteoporotic fracture in one part of your body, you are more likely to suffer another fracture in another area, osteoporosis being progressive and capable of inflicting several disabilities.

Management of the problem

Careful management under your doctor's supervision can probably reduce the rate of further bone loss, possibly stop loss of bone and even gradually strengthen your skeletal mass.

If you have secondary osteoporosis due to another disease or condition, treatment of this other ailment early enough to save your bone mass can be beneficial. If, for instance, you can reduce your need for drugs to combat inflammatory arthritis, or hyperthyroidism, you may be able to prevent the loss to your skeleton that these can cause, apart from age-related bone loss. Here are further useful ideas for your fight against osteoporosis:

1. Have regular bone-density tests performed by your personal physician or at your local clinic, every three to six months

depending on severity, so your skeletal mass can be monitored.

2. Eliminate as many 'negative factors' as you can (e.g., stop or cut down smoking and drinking) and 'accentuate the positive' (e.g., eat well, drink plenty of lowfat milk, get as much exercise as you can manage, and be out in the sunshine!).

3. Keep a daily log of dietary calcium and vitamins and other supplements (perhaps utilizing your home computer). Calcium should be at least 1200 to 1500 mg each day.

4. Check that your bed is comfortable with firm support; a sheet of ¾ in (2 cm) plywood beneath the mattress is an instant and inexpensive solution, or try a water bed.

5. Immediately after back injury, or when you have strained muscles, ice packs will help reduce swelling and inflammation. Rest as much as you can.

6. If your back problem is stiffness on waking, try warmth to soothe and relax: a warm bath, the warm sun, warm heating pads.

7. Massage can increase the flow of blood to your back and relax muscles.

8. Gentle stretching exercises can flex your back muscles; swimming can give you gentle exercise while supporting your body.

9. Prolonged sitting can place more stress on your back than standing, since your pelvis is not supporting you in that position. Change positions often, whether in bed, at home, or at work, and be sure your chair has a back-rest, preferably adjustable.

10. Women should look critically at the heel height of their shoes and discard any pair with heels of more than 1½ in.

11. Use painkillers sparingly – they can be addictive, and if pain is masked, you could further injure your back unknowingly.

Prevention of accidents that may cause fracturing

1. Have a good supportive pillow (perhaps a water pillow) to support your neck vertebrae. Sometimes a low pillow will let the spine become an unsupported arch, sagging under its own weight, allowing vertebrae to rub against each other. The

first symptom will usually be neck pain on waking.

2. Learn to lift heavy objects properly, *bending your knees* so that you use the strength of your legs and do not strain your back. A major reason for small fractures of the spine associated with osteoporosis is unnecessary bending from the waist.

3. Remember simple tools like long-handled shoe horns to minimize awkward bending.

4. All small rugs and carpet edges should be secured down to the floor.

5. Floors should not be highly polished.

6. Wipe up all spills from kitchen and bathroom floors immediately.

7. Make sure electrical wires are not trailing across rooms where they could be tripped over.

8. When buying slippers, choose those with soles that grip well for a firm footing.

9. If children are in the house, be careful of toys left on the floor.

10. Install grab bars on the side of the bath or beside the shower, to ease getting in and out.

11. Install non-slip strips in the bottom of the bath or shower.

12. Install non-slip strips on indoor or outdoor steps, on stepladders and walkways.

13. Plug in tiny night-lights in hallways or bathrooms to avoid stumbling in the dark.

14. Never stand on chairs or stacks of books to reach high shelves. Have a small stepladder handy, or buy pick-up tongs from a mail-order company, for hard-to-reach items.

15. Water high-up house plants with a water-wand; wash second-storey windows with a hose extension.

16. Install rails or banisters to all stairs.

17. Be sure spectacles are clean, so that dust specks don't create distractions. If a new prescription for glasses causes problems, see your opthalmologist promptly. Take extra care when wearing bifocals.

18. In the garden, never leave hoses or tools on the ground where they could be tripped over; hang them up when not in use.

19. Have good lighting on paths and driveways, and keep ice and snow cleared. Be wary of uneven or slippery kerbs.

20. When shopping, use a trolley for support, even if only buying a few items.

Safety with medicines and supplements

We live at a time when science is pursuing so many fields of research, and in the medical field so many more drugs and medications are available to improve our health. The growth of our population over the age of sixty-five can be due at least in part, to the availability of effective medicines and vaccines. The D.H.S.S. reports that during 1984 as many as 53 per cent of prescriptions dispensed in England were for women over the age of sixty and for men over sixty-five. Of course, it is only natural that older people have more long-term illnesses (such as arthritis, heart disease and hypertension). And it is not uncommon to have a number of disabilities or diseases at the same time for which you need to take a number of different medications. But have we become an over-medicated society?

Generally speaking, the elderly can have different reactions to medicines than the young or middle-aged, probably because of the decrease in the percentage of lean tissue (including muscle) and an increase in the percentage of fat. Consequently, these differences can affect the drug amount that is absorbed by body tissues and the length of time it remains in the body. Older people seem to have more undesirable reactions to drugs than younger people, probably because organs like the kidneys and the liver are working less efficiently, so that drugs (including alcohol) are slower to leave the body.

Prescription drugs are generally more powerful and may have more side reactions than over-the-counter medicines; and yet when large quantities of non-prescription drugs are taken, if they have strong ingredients, they might equal or exceed a dose available in a prescription. Some medicines (including antacids, alcohol, cold remedies, laxatives and vitamins) can create difficulties if over-used or abused or taken in combination with prescription drugs, causing dizziness or drowsiness that could result in stumbling or falling. These few basic rules can help you use medicines, mineral and vitamin supplements more safely:

1. Before you have a new prescription, tell your doctor all the

other medicines you are taking, including oral contraceptives, insulin, non-prescription drugs and those prescribed by other doctors, plus vitamin and mineral supplements. If you are pregnant, a heavy smoker, or a heavy drinker, ask your doctor if there are any special foods, alcohol or aspirin to avoid, and if medicines should be with or between meals. Ask specifically what effect the new medication will have on your bone mineralization (especially if it is cortisone, an anti-coagulant, anticonvulsant, tranquillizer or stimulant), and if additional calcium or vitamin supplements may be necessary.

2. Tell your doctor about previous adverse reactions you have had with medications (dizziness, rashes, indigestion, constipation, etc.). Know exactly what the medication is supposed to do for you, and ask about any side effects that may occur with a new prescription. Phone your doctor immediately if you have unusual effects.

3. Understand exactly what the dosage should be and how frequent, and take precisely the dosage your doctor prescribes. Oral contraceptives, oestrogens and a few other drugs usually have an information leaflet detailing risks and benefits. Read this brochure carefully.

4. Never take medicines prescribed for a relative or friend, or give your medication to anyone else, even though you may have similar symptoms or illness. Medicines can produce different effects in everyone.

5. Make a complete daily record of each drug and supplement you are taking, particularly if you are taking more than one. Note the name of the drug, the amount you take and the times of day for the dose, and don't forget to tick off each dose as you take it.

6. Ask the chemist for easy-to-open containers if child-proof tops are difficult for you. Be sure to keep all medicines and supplements locked up and well out of the reach of children. Ask the pharmacist about any special storage requirements for the medicines you take, such as refrigeration.

7. Ask your chemist to put large type on the medicine label if you find the usual type difficult to read. Make sure you have the name of the medicine clearly on the label with the dosage

directions, and that you understand them. If you have any doubt that they are different from what your doctor has told you, mention this to your pharmacist or doctor.

8. Never put medicines into unlabelled containers. Fancy pill boxes are not always suitable.

9. Never take medicines at night without turning on the light. Be sure you can see clearly what you are taking and how much.

10. If you feel a medicine may be doing you more harm than good, don't stop taking it without asking your doctor; he may want to change the dosage or substitute another medication that is more suitable to your changing needs.

11. Never resume taking a drug you happen to have in the medicine cabinet without checking with your doctor.

12. Many medications lose their strength and effectiveness over a period of time, so expiry dates should be carefully checked. Old medicines should be cautiously discarded and the labels clearly marked 'Empty' (to give peace of mind if children are found playing with the old jars or bottles).

Chapter 10
A QUICK A TO Z GUIDE TO GOOD BONE BUILDING

Alcohol. If you drink to excess, it may affect the ability of your liver to activate vitamin D; it may impair the absorption of calcium through your intestines. It's not the type of beverage, but the amount of alcohol in it. Many drugs and mouthwashes also contain alcohol.

Almonds. Good for bone building but caloric. Have unsalted whole almonds for snacks. Use almond paste for biscuits and homemade sweets.

Aluminium. Avoid antacids containing aluminium and sodium. Read labels carefully and change to brands with calcium. Avoid drinking water clarified with aluminium salts. Discard worn and pitted aluminium cookware.

Anticonvulsant drugs. Special care has to be taken to maintain calcium intake when these drugs are prescribed by your doctor. You may need to change drugs or the brand of your prescription.

Beans. Canned beans are usually high-sodium and best avoided by good bone builders. Cook dried beans 'from scratch' in unsalted water and no bicarbonate of soda. Beans, in combination with rice or pasta or corn tortillas, can make a good contribution to your protein intake, and reduce your consumption of red meats.

Beet greens. Best avoided in large amounts by bone builders because of the oxalic acid they contain that can lead to calcium depletion.

Bicycling. Good exercise for the cardiovascular system, and the promotion of strong muscles and bones.

Bones. Chop or mash the soft bones of canned salmon and canned sardines to include in dishes to maximize the calcium content.

Bran. Large amounts of raw bran are to be avoided because of the phytic acid which binds with calcium to reduce absorption.

Breads and flours. Choose wholewheat and fortified types whenever possible to maximize calcium content.

Breakfast cereals. Enrich cooked cereals by stirring in powdered skimmed milk and sweetening with molasses or dark treacle.

Broccoli. A good source of calcium. Cook in unsalted water.

Butter. To boost calcium and reduce calories (because of doubled volume), whip ½ cup butter or margarine with ¼ cup skimmed milk.

Buttermilk. A good source of calcium, often tolerated when plain milk cannot be. Use in pancake and waffle batters, mixed half and half with mayonnaise for fresh, tangy salad dressings, enhanced with your own herbs. Create beverages with buttermilk plus your choice of pineapple, grape or tomato juice, puréed strawberries or peaches. Combine buttermilk with eggs, ice-milk, vanilla and a sprinkle of cinnamon for a nourishing nog-type drink. Tenderize pot roasts with a buttermilk marinade. For a chilled soup, blend buttermilk, egg yolks, sugar, lemon juice, grated lemon rind and vanilla.

Caffeine. Moderation! Excessive drinking of coffee, tea, cocoa, soft drinks, can rob your body of calcium. Alternatives are herbal teas (although not in large quantities). Use carob instead of cocoa and chocolate; natural fresh fruit juices instead of soft cola drinks. Ask your doctor or pharmacist for medicine without caffeine.

Calcium. The cornerstone of good bone building. Your body depends on you to supply daily needs. You never outgrow your need for calcium. Best sources are milk, yogurt, cheeses, canned salmon and sardines.

Calcium supplements. Calcium is best obtained from good nutrition.

But when dairy products are not tolerated, soya substitutes unacceptable, and calcium poorly absorbed, supplements can be helpful. Calcium carbonate found in some antacid remedies is the cheapest form of supplement, but excess can cause constipation or stomach irritation. Several other supplements are available, including bone meal, but this latter may have an excessive lead content.

Carob. To avoid caffeine in chocolate, use carob as a substitute, as in carob milk, carob ice cream and carob powder for baking.

Cheeses. Excellent concentrated sources of calcium and the other nutrients found in milk, with hundreds of varieties to choose from. Some are more digestible than others, and some have a higher calcium content (e.g., Cheddar, Edam, Gouda). Avoid higher-sodium cheeses such as Roquefort, blue, Féta and Stilton. Add cheese to salads, casseroles. Sprinkle on soups. Vegetables can be accented with cheese sauce or a sprinkling of grated cheese. Use Parmesan cheese instead of salt. Add cheese to pie-crusts, hot popcorn; sprinkle small Cheddar dice into casseroles and potato salad. Cheese makes economical main dishes: quiche lorraine, lasagne, omelettes. Cheddar, mozzarella and Edam cheeses freeze well, as an emergency supply.

Chocolate. If you have a sweet tooth, turn to carob instead, to reduce caffeine intake and boost calcium.

Cigarettes. Smoking is robbing you of bone tissue. Cut down or cut out entirely.

Coffee. Drink in moderation to avoid caffeine and phytate. Avoid non-dairy creamers, that can increase sodium and not calcium.

Collards. A good source of calcium. Cook in unsalted water. Season with nutmeg or other herbs for variety and intriguing flavour.

Cream and sour cream. Good sources of calcium, but because of high fat content you may want to limit intake to keep cholesterol and calories low. Substitute lowfat yogurt on baked potatoes or fruit. For a low-calorie whipped topping, chill ⅓ cup dry nonfat milk, ½ cup water and 1 tablespoon lemon juice. Beat well and sweeten to taste.

Dieting. Slimming diets can be hazardous and create bone loss unless adequate calcium and vitamins are included.

Diuretics. These drugs for increasing urine may contribute to calcium loss. Thiazides would be more suitable for older women.

Dried milk. Nonfat dried milk is a handy way to take calcium, without adding fat to your diet and consequent calories. Dried milk can be added to soups, casseroles and many other dishes to give added calcium value.

Eggs. Instead of frying eggs, scramble them with skimmed milk to increase calcium value.

Exercise. Should be part of every day and part of your lifestyle. There are many different levels of activity, depending on your current state of health. Even the bedridden can perform certain movements, to help stimulate blood circulation and tone up the system, maintaining calcium balance. Most beneficial is daily walking, regular swimming, cycling, stretching and light tennis. Let exercise be *fun*, to help you do it regularly.

Fats and oils. Reduce fat consumption for a healthy heart, but without sacrifice of calcium for strong bones: remember dairy products such as skimmed milk and lowfat cheeses.

Fibre. Part of a good all-round diet, but too much bran can sweep food through your digestive tract without absorption of nutrients in your intestines. Phytic acid, in the outer husks of cereal grains, can combine with calcium in your digestive system and reduce calcium absorption. Better alternatives for adding bulk would be leafy green vegetables, fresh whole fruits and wholegrain breads every day.

Fluoride. Fluoride is present naturally in drinking water in most areas, but some communities have increased the natural level in order to reduce tooth decay, strengthen tooth enamel and bones. Excessive amounts can cause mottling of teeth and may harm the kidneys. Fluoride is also present in minute quantities in some foods.

Gelatine. One tablespoon of unflavoured gelatine is only 25 calories. Stir into homemade soups and stews to enrich collagen in your connective tissues. Make your own varieties of jellies for desserts using fresh fruit juices or lowfat milk.

Goat's milk. A good source of calcium if cow's milk is not available or not digestible. However, it is higher in saturated fat.

Gum disease. Can be an early warning of lack of calcium or vitamin C and a sign of bone demineralization – or poor dental hygiene. Daily brushing and flossing of teeth is essential, along with proper intake of calcium and vitamin C.

Herbs. Use liberally to season foods, to replace salt, but add variety and flavour interest.

Ice-cream and ice-milk. A delicious way to take calcium, and so many different flavours to choose! Ice-milk is a good way to have your dessert without extra calories found in ice-cream. Serve over fresh, canned or stewed fruit, over waffles, between nut-bread slices, blended in milk-shakes or floated on chocolate milk.

Indigestion remedies. Avoid antacids containing aluminium. Some remedies contain calcium and can be used as supplements.

Jogging. As part of a health programme of exercise, jogging can be beneficial, but have a thorough check with your doctor before starting a new vigorous form of exercise. Not for those who already have porous or brittle bones.

Juices. For a healthy supply of vitamins, choose fruit juices and not fruit drinks or fruit-flavoured soft drinks.

Kidney stones. Can be a problem for some people, in which case calcium would need to be reduced. This painful condition is generally hereditary, sometimes caused by excess intake of calcium, vitamins, reduced intake of liquids, reduced exercise, or other metabolic disturbances.

Lactase. An enzyme in your digestive tract that helps the digestion of milk and dairy products. If you are deficient in lactase, supplements may be taken in drop form or tablets, to add to milk.

Laxatives. Over-use of laxatives can result in poor absorption of calcium, with consequent bone depletion. Improve your diet, drink more liquids and get more exercise, to tone up your system.

Lettuce. The greener the lettuce leaf, the richer in calcium, and vitamins A and C.

Meat. Too much red meat, with an intake of too much protein and phosphorus, can cause your body to lose calcium. Use more vegetable protein combinations, casseroles, poultry, fish and lowfat dairy produce.

Milk. High-quality protein, and an excellent source of calcium for bone building. Waist-watchers choose lowfat or skimmed milk. If digesting milk is a problem, drink it warmed, or add one of the enzyme lactase supplements. Always have fresh milk on hand, and powdered, canned or evaporated milk on your pantry shelf. Prepare canned soups and chowders with milk instead of water. Put milk into puddings and macaroni cheese, cream sauces, cereals cooked with milk, custards, cocoa made with milk, milk-shakes and party punches. When necessary, milk can be frozen: its consistency will change, but not its nutrition. Thaw in the refrigerator and stir occasionally. Extend shelf-life of milk by microwaving on full power for two minutes in small quantities of about 1 cup at a time. Carefully read labels of imitation milk. You could be shortchanged on calcium while increasing unwanted sodium, sugar and calories.

Molasses. Use molasses or dark treacle instead of sugar to sweeten cooked cereals, cakes and biscuits, to flavour plain yogurt and milk-shakes, and in toffee-making.

Non-dairy creamers. Check the labels of powdered or liquid coffee creamers. Non-dairy products have little calcium value, and much saturated fat derived from coconut oil is used in processing.

Nuts and seeds. Good sources of calcium for bone building, but the oils in them can make them caloric. Choose almonds, hazelnuts, peanuts with skins left on, and either whole, slivered, chopped or made into pastes and butters. Choose unsalted nut snacks for reduced sodium.

Oestrogen Replacement Therapy. Can prevent bone loss caused by natural menopause or surgical removal of your ovaries, but there are risks and it is still considered somewhat controversial unless progestin is taken in conjunction with oestrogen.

Oral contraceptives. If approved by your doctor, these drugs can help you maintain and strengthen your bone density, but they do carry certain risks.

Oranges and other citrus. For vitamin C, important in bone formation, be sure to have ½ cup of orange juice or a whole orange every day.

Oxalates. Oxalic acid. Natural compounds that interfere with calcium absorption, found in some green leafy vegetables, such as beet greens, silverbeet, spinach and also in rhubarb.

Pasta. Combine with peas, beans, lentils or tofu, to make good protein without red meat.

Phosphorus. The ratio of phosphorus to calcium should be about 1:1. Too much phosphorus can deplete the body of calcium. Avoid red meats, cola drinks and brewer's yeast, and processed foods that have large amounts of phosphorus.

Phytates. Phosphorus-containing natural compounds interfering with calcium absorption, and found in the outer husk of cereal grains, and in strong infusions of tea, coffee and cocoa. Phytates are sometimes referred to as phytic acid.

Protein. Large servings of red-meat protein can deplete your body of calcium. Although protein is one of the building-blocks of your body, needs can be met with combinations of rice/peas, rice/beans, wheat/peanuts, etc.

Rhubarb. It's healthy to eat a variety of foods for good nutrition, but since rhubarb is high in oxalic acid it can rob your body of calcium if eaten in excessive amounts.

Salad dressings and mayonnaise. Thin with nonfat plain yogurt when possible. Choose cheese-type dressings instead of oil and vinegar.

Salmon. Use canned salmon, drained of its liquid, but with the bones chopped in for a good calcium source. Make salmon spreads for appetizers, fill small pastry cases for cocktail puffs, stir into chicken broth to make soup or chowder, use in salads and sandwiches seasoned with lemon juice and herbs. Salmon is good in casseroles, creamed dishes and salmon loaf.

Salt and sodium. With too much salt and sodium in your diet, you lose more calcium. Apart from not using the salt cellar, avoid canned processed foods that are high in sodium, monosodium glutamate, soya sauce, Worcestershire sauce, ham, bacon, anchovies, salted cured fish, olives and pickles.

Sardines. Canned sardines with bones included, are good bone builders. Choose sardines canned in water or in tomato sauce. Sardines in oils are high in fat and should be avoided for a healthy heart. Serve sardines often – as appetizers, in salads and sandwiches, on pizza or in a casserole with potatoes au gratin.

Silverbeet. Silverbeet (or Swiss chard) in vast amounts is best avoided for good bone building, because of its oxalic acid content. Serve other leafy green vegetables, such as collards or broccoli.

Smoking. A 'bone robber'. Cut it out, or cut it down.

Soft drinks. Cut out or reduce your consumption of soft drinks containing large amounts of phosphorus, to keep a better calcium-phosphorus ratio.

Sour cream. A source of calcium, but also high in fat. Substitute lowfat plain yogurt on potatoes or in recipes whenever possible.

Soya products. When cow's milk and dairy products are not easily digested, turn to soya bean products. Look for calcium-fortified soya milk. Soya powder can be used for making a milk-substitute; tofu can substitute for dairy products. But avoid miso which is high-sodium. Toss tofu cubes into salads and soups; blend with fruit for desserts; blend with oil, vinegar and minced onion for a thick salad dressing or dip. Tofu can substitute for cheese or meat in entrées, casseroles, omelettes and cheesecake.

Spinach. High in oxalic acid that can interfere with calcium absorption, so large amounts are best avoided for good bone building.

Stress. Can stimulate adrenal hormones that cause bone depletion. Relax, exercise, or accept the situation that is causing your problems.

Sugars. Cut down or cut out to control weight and improve dental hygiene. If you must have sugar, use brown in place of white whenever possible, or sweeten dishes with dark treacle, to enhance calcium intake.

Sunshine. Free vitamin D comes to you from sunshine by the action of ultraviolet light on your skin. Try to get daily amounts of sunshine, without overdoing it and getting sunburned. With this free vitamin D, you absorb more calcium in foods. You need the ultraviolet light gained from being outdoors, not just in a sunny window where the rays can't penetrate the glass. Vitamin D tablets or drops are available free or at a reduced price, if you are pregnant or have young babies. Overdose of vitamin D can cause bone loss.

Swimming. A good form of exercise for firming muscles and keeping bones healthy, even if you already have osteoporosis.

Tea. Use in moderation, to avoid caffeine and phytate. Take tea with milk instead of a lemon slice. Avoid non-dairy creamers with no calcium.

Thyroid supplements. These drugs can contribute to calcium loss. Check dosage with your doctor.

Tofu. A thick firm curd made from soya beans, long used in the Far East where milk is not easily digested, it has now been introduced to the Western diet. It's a good calcium source. Try it!

Tortillas. Choose corn tortillas rather than flour tortillas, as lime is used to process corn during manufacture, increasing calcium. One tortilla has 60 mg of calcium. Make quesadillas: sprinkle corn tortillas with Cheddar, then slip under the grill for a few minutes.

Turnip greens. High in oxalic acid, and to be avoided by bone builders.

Vegetables. Have generous servings of fresh vegetables every day for a healthy intake of calcium and vitamins, plus fibre for promoting regularity without laxatives. Green leaf vegetables provide vitamin C; yellow vegetables have vitamin A. Don't use salt for washing or cooking vegetables. Steam or cook lightly to preserve nutrients. Enhance flavours with a variety of herbs or spices.

Vegetarianism. Provided that plenty of dairy products are included, vegetarianism can be conducive to good bone formation.

Vitamins. Apart from calcium, the heroes for bone builders are vitamins D, A and C. Vitamin deficiency can cause bone depletion; but overdose can be toxic or trigger bone loss. Get vitamin D from daily sunshine and fortified margarine; vitamin A is in fortified margarine, yellow fruits and vegetables; vitamin C is in citrus juices and fruits and green leafy vegetables.

Walking. Walk daily, instead of jumping into the car for errands. You need regular exercise for muscle tone and strong bones. Walking can be done by almost everyone and it's free!

Water supply. Check your household water supply for levels of calcium, fluoride and sodium. Calcium and fluoride in water help to build strong bones and teeth. Sodium can deplete your bone level. Be sure your water conditioner is not extracting the nutrients you need.

Weight control. Try to avoid sudden increases in weight that can strain already weakened bones.

White sauce, 'cream' sauce. Made with nonfat milk, these sauces can add calcium value to vegetables, casseroles, fish, poultry and eggs.

X-rays. Useful tools for measuring bone density, and your susceptibility to osteoporosis.

Yeast. Avoid excessive amounts of brewer's yeast (such as in beers) because of the high proportion of phosphorus in relation to calcium.

Yogurt. When you can't digest milk easily, try yogurt, with meals or as a snack, avoiding flavoured sweetened yogurts; lowfat or nonfat will have fewer calories. Unflavoured yogurt can be delicious with fresh fruit, a small spoonful of preserves, molasses or treacle, or a dash of spice. Live-cultured yogurt will benefit your intestinal tract. Substitute plain yogurt for sour cream on mashed or baked potatoes, with or without chives. Use half yogurt, half mayonnaise, for a tangy salad dressing or topping for vegetables or fruits. Serve yogurt over ready-prepared cereal. Substitute 1 cup of yogurt for 1 cup of cold water when making jelly desserts. Serve yogurt and fruit in layers in parfait glasses.

Zinc, Lead, Cadmium, Mercury. Toxic particles of matter in pollution that can affect your bone mass when calcium intake is low.

THE LAST WORD

A sixteenth-century herbal says 'Give him a drinke of Cumphorie (comfrey) hearbe stamped with milk or ale, for that will helpe to knit the bones.'

We now have the benefit of modern medicine, advanced research and 'high-tech' diagnostic techniques. Osteoporosis is a sad deforming, crippling bone disease, slowly developing and now reaching the proportions of an epidemic among older people, especially women, with an enormous impact of physical suffering, emotional strain and financial hardship. There is no cure, and once bone is lost it cannot be regained; but as more aspects of prevention and treatment of this disease become known, future generations may be spared this terrible suffering.

Meanwhile, much can be done with a lifelong course of preventive action against osteoporosis, beginning early in life with sufficient intake of calcium-rich foods such as milk and dairy products together with regular daily exercise. Good nutrition and healthy physical activity can go a long way to strengthen bones to last you a lifetime. Making your bones dense and stronger *now* will reduce your risk of osteoporosis in ten–twenty–thirty years' time. True health insurance is what you do for yourself. You expect your bones to support *you* for the rest of your life – do as much as you can to support *them*.

Appendix I
DAILY NUTRITION CHART FOR GOOD BONE BUILDING

Nutrients	Average adult		Women over 55	Pregnant		Nursing	
	Men[a]	Women[a]		under 18	over 18	under 18	over 18
Energy (calories)	2825	2150	1900	2400	2400	2750	2750
Protein (g)	70	54	47	60	60	69	69
Calcium (mg)[b]	1000	1000	1500	1500[c]	1200	1500[c]	1200
Vit. A (μg)	750	750	750	750	750	1200	1200
Vit. C (mg)	30	30	30	60	60	60	60
Vit. D (μg)	_[d]	_[d]	_[d]	10	10	10	10
Fat (g)[e]	94	72	63	80	80	92	92
Sodium (mg)[f]	2000 max.	2000 max.	2000 max.	2000 max.	2000 max.	2000 max.	2000 max.

a Moderately active.
b Recommendation of the National Osteoporosis Society. Calcium for women to be 1500mg between the ages of 40 and 60.
c This figure represents 300mg more than the needs of a non-pregnant girl.
d The housebound and the elderly during winter need 10 micrograms.
e Calories derived from fat should equal 30 per cent of total
f Recommendation of World Health Organization and the American Heart Association.

Appendix II

GLOSSARY OF MEDICAL TERMS

Adenosis. A condition seen mostly in daughters exposed to DES (Diethylstilbesterol). Patches of mucus-secreting cells on the cervix or vaginal wall.

Adrenal glands. Small, pyramid-shaped, located close to the kidneys.

Adrenal hormones. Made and released by the adrenals. Some adrenal hormones are harmful to bone remodelling.

Adrenopause. Around the age of sixty-five, when some adrenal production slows.

Alveolar bone. Section of jaw containing the tooth sockets.

Amenorrhoeic. Without menstrual periods.

Anabolic steroids. Growth hormones, similar to androgens.

Androgens. Male hormones, produced by men's testes and adrenals, and by women's adrenals and ovaries in small amounts. Responsible for the appearance of pubic and underarm hair.

Anticoagulants. Drugs used to thin blood to control heart disease.

Anticonvulsants. Drugs used to control epileptic seizures.

Bone mass. Total amount of bone in the body. Overall, it increases from birth to around the age of thirty, and thereafter is lost with age.

Calcitonin. Hormone released mostly by the thyroid gland. It slows down bone loss.

Calcium. Metallic element in nearly all living tissue. It gives bone its structural properties. 99 per cent of the body's calcium is in the bones. Calcium is required for muscle contraction, normal blood clotting and nerves.

Calipers. An instrument with two curved legs used to make fine measurements.

CAT scan. Computerized Axial Tomography, used to view tissue or bone in a cross section by X-ray.

Cervix. The narrowing lower end ('neck') of the uterus from where Pap smears are taken.

Climacteric. Change of life. Ovarian function decreases and eventually ceases entirely.

Cod-fishing. Collapse of two spinal vertebrae, so the space between looks fish-shaped.

Collagen. Protein that supports bone, cartilage, skin and connective tissue.

Colles fracture. Wrist fracture involving the end of the radius bone.

Corpus luteum. A small gland located in the ovary producing progesterone after ovulation. If conception occurs, the gland also makes the hormones necessary to support pregnancy for the first few months.

Cortical bone. Hard outer bone surrounding trabecular bone material.

Corticosteroids. Drugs sometimes used to treat arthritis or asthma. They resemble adrenal hormones.

Cortisone. An adrenal hormone that can be harmful to bone. It also can be a drug resembling the adrenal hormone.

Crush fracture. A vertebra that has collapsed completely.

D and C. Dilation and curettage. The procedure of a physician for opening the entry to the uterus and scraping away the uterus lining (endometrium), for diagnosis or therapy.

Densitometer. An instrument used to measure the density of bones by the amount of radiation they absorb.

Diethylstilbesterol (DES). A synthetic oestrogen widely used in the 1940s to help maintain a pregnancy – later proved ineffective. Nowadays it is known that DES could have many harmful effects. Daughters exposed to DES have a greater risk of vaginal cancer and adenosis, and reduced fertility; sons exposed to DES may develop abnormalities of the genitals and reduced fertility.

Diuretics. Drugs used to increase the production of urine.

Dual photon absorptiometry. A sensitive method of measuring spinal bone.

Endometrium. The lining part of the uterus.

Femur. Thigh bone.

Fibroid uterine tumour. A non-malignant growth of the uterine muscle. Small fibroids often are without symptoms. When symptoms are present they may include prolonged menstruation, frequent urination or bleeding between menstrual periods.

Follicle. A small sac in the ovary containing the developing egg and lined by special cells that produce oestrogen and progesterone. After ovulation, the sac becomes the corpus luteum.

Growth hormone. Produced by the pituitary gland to promote tissue growth.

Hormone Replacement Therapy (HRT). Usually including progestin as well as oestrogen, often prescibed following surgical or natural menopause to supplement hormones.

Hypercalciuria. Excessive excretion of calcium in the urine.

Hysterectomy. The surgical removal of the uterus. Total or complete hysterectomy means the removal of uterus and cervix, plus ovaries. Subtotal hysterectomy is the removal of the uterus but not the cervix.

Hysteroscopy. A diagnostic procedure, usually under anaesthesia, in which a viewing instrument (hysteroscope) is inserted in the uterus to detect disease.

Kyphosis. Abnormal curvature of the upper spine, leading to a 'dowager's hump'.

Lactase. An enzyme in the intestines that digests lactose mostly found in milk products.

Lactase deficiency. A shortage of lactase that causes stomach discomfort when lactose is eaten.

Lactose. 'Milk sugar', a sugar naturally occurring in milk and dairy produce. Also used in some baby foods, baked goods, sweets and medicines.

Lactose intolerance. See 'Lactase deficiency'.

Lordosis. Abnormal inward curving of the lower spine.

Menarche. Beginning of menstrual periods at puberty.

Natural menopause. A phase in women, with decreased oestrogen and progesterone production, the cessation of menstrual periods, and the inability to bear children. The average menopausal age for European and American women is about fifty. A woman in this age range who has not menstruated for a year is said to have passed into menopause.

Natural oestrogens. Oestrogens that are the same chemically as those occurring in nature, often obtained from animal sources.

Nulliparous. Never having borne a child.

Oestrogen. Female hormone produced by ovaries in women and in small quantities by male testes. Oestrogens stimulate the development of cervical mucus and ovulation, and help prepare the uterine lining for possible implantation after conception. Laboratory-produced oestrogens can correct hormonal problems.

Oestrogen Replacement Therapy. More recently referred to as Hormone Replacement Therapy, whereby hormones are prescribed following surgical or natural menopause. It may increase the risk of uterine cancer as much as seven-fold.

Oophorectomy. Surgical removal of the ovaries.

Osteoblasts. Bone-making cells.

Osteoclasts. Cells that resorb and dissolve bone tissue.

Osteomalacia. Adult disease of under-mineralized bone resulting from a deficiency of vitamin D. In children this disease is referred to as rickets.

Osteopenia. A below-normal level of bone mass.

Osteoporosis. Abnormal porosity and thinning of bones, with a reduction of bone mass, leading to easily fractured bones.

Ovariectomy. See 'Oophorectomy'.

Ovary. One of two organs in women containing the cells which produce the female hormones oestrogen and progesterone (and small amounts of the masculine hormone androgen). Ovaries contain a woman's lifetime supply of eggs, generally depleted by menopause.

Oxalates. Oxalic acid. Natural compounds found in some leafy green vegetables; e.g., spinach, beet greens, silverbeet. Also found in rhubarb. When eaten in excessive amounts, these compounds can interfere with calcium absorption.

Parathyroid. Four small organs near the thyroid.

Parathyroid hormone. Released by the parathyroid glands in response to low blood-calcium, triggering bone breakdown to transfer calcium to the bloodstream.

Periodontal disease. Gum inflammation in tooth-supporting tissues, loosening teeth.

Phosphorus. A non-metallic element in all living tissues, involved with metabolism. It constitutes part of your bone structure, with calcium.

Phytates. Phytic acid. Natural compounds containing phosphorus interfering with calcium absorption when eaten in excessive amounts. Phytates are in the outer husks of cereal grains, tea leaves, coffee beans and cacao seeds, and other plant material.

Pituitary gland. Situated at the base of the brain, this gland produces many hormones.

Progesterone. A multi-purpose hormone produced primarily by the corpus luteum after ovulation, during the second half of the menstrual cycle. Small amounts are also produced by the adrenal cortex. The hormone inhibits further ovulations and helps prepare the uterus to nourish the embryo after implantation.

Progestogen or Progestin. A synthetic hormone similar to progesterone.

Prolactin. A hormone produced by the pituitary gland, stimulating milk production (lactation) after childbirth.

Pyorrhoea. Gum disease. See 'Periodontal disease'.

Radiographic photodensitometry. A method to measure bone density by X-rays.

Radius. The smaller of the two bones in the forearm.

Resorption. The breakdown and dissolving of bone in the process of remodelling.

Single photon absorptiometry. A method to measure density of long bones.

Sodium. An element found in table salt (as sodium chloride), and many foods and drugs.

Surgical menopause. Surgical removal of ovaries prior to natural menopause.

Synthetic oestrogens. Oestrogens differing chemically from those occurring in nature.

Thyroid gland. Organ at the base of the neck controlling the metabolic rate.

Trabecular bone. The inner honeycomb-like bone tissue, surrounded by the more dense cortical bone material.

Ulna. The larger of the two bones in the forearm.

Uterus. The womb.

Wedge fracture. Fracture occurring in one of the spinal vertebrae.

Appendix III

CALCIUM, PHOSPHORUS AND CALORIE CONTENT OF COMMON FOODS

Item	Food	Amount	Ca (mg)	P (mg)	Calories
DAIRY PRODUCTS					
Milk					
1.	Cow's, fresh whole	150ml/¼pt	180	142	98
2.	skimmed	150ml/¼pt	195	150	50
3.	sterilized and longlife	150ml/¼pt	180	142	98
4.	condensed, whole, sweetened	150ml/¼pt	420	330	483
5.	condensed, skimmed, sweetened	150ml/¼pt	570	405	400
6.	evaporated, whole, unsweetened	150ml/¼pt	420	375	237
7.	dried, skimmed	100g/3½oz	1190	950	355
8.	Goat's	150ml/¼pt	195	165	106
9.	Human (10 days after birth)	150ml/¼pt	37	24	100
10.	(1 month after birth)	150ml/¼pt	51	21	103
Milk Desserts					
11.	Egg custard	100g/3½oz	130	140	118
12.	Ice-cream, dairy	100g/3½oz	140	100	167
13.	Jelly made with milk	100g/3½oz	59	42	86
14.	Milk pudding	100g/3½oz	130	110	131
15.	Yogurt, natural	100g/3½oz	180	140	52
16.	flavoured	100g/3½oz	170	140	81

Item	Food	Amount	Ca (mg)	P (mg)	Calories
17.	fruit	100g/3½oz	160	140	95
Cream					
18.	Cream, single	100g/3½oz	79	44	212
19.	double	100g/3½oz	50	21	447
20.	whipping	100g/3½oz	63	27	332
21.	sterilized, canned	100g/3½oz	80	44	230
Cheese, natural					
22.	Camembert type	50g/2oz	190	145	150
23.	Cheddar type	50g/2oz	400	260	203
24.	Danish Blue type	50g/2oz	290	215	177
25.	Edam type	50g/2oz	370	260	152
26.	Féta	50g/2oz	192	n/a	122
27.	Parmesan, grated	25g/1oz	305	192	102
28.	Stilton (blue)	50g/2oz	180	150	231
Cheese, processed					
29.	Cheese spread	50g/2oz	255	220	141
30.	Cottage	100g/3½oz	60	140	96
31.	Cream cheese	50g/2oz	49	50	219
32.	Processed	50g/2oz	350	245	155
Cheese dishes					
33.	Cauliflower cheese	100g/3½oz	160	120	113
34.	Cheese soufflé	100g/3½oz	230	230	252
35.	Macaroni cheese	100g/3½oz	180	140	174
36.	Pizza (cheese and tomato)	100g/3½oz	240	170	234
37.	Quiche Lorraine	100g/3½oz	260	240	391
38.	Welsh rarebit	100g/3½oz	420	290	365
Eggs					
39.	Raw, whole, large	1 egg	26	110	73
40.	Scrambled with milk	1 egg	30	95	123

FISH, MEAT, POULTRY AND RELATED PRODUCTS

Item	Food	Amount	Ca (mg)	P (mg)	Calories
Fish					
41.	Cod, fried in batter	100g/3½oz	80	200	199
42.	Haddock, fried	100g/3½oz	110	250	174

Item	Food	Amount	Ca (mg)	P (mg)	Calories
43.	Halibut, steamed	100g/3½oz	13	260	131
44.	Lemon sole, steamed	100g/3½oz	21	250	91
45.	Plaice, fried in batter	100g/3½oz	93	170	279
46.	Salmon, pink, canned (including bones)	100g/3½oz	195	283	140
47.	Sardines, canned in oil	100g/3½oz	460	430	334
48.	Sardines, canned in tomato sauce	100g/3½oz	460	400	177
49.	Tuna, canned in oil	100g/3½oz	7	190	289
Shellfish					
50.	Crab, boiled	100g/3½oz	29	350	127
51.	Lobster, boiled	100g/3½oz	62	280	119
52.	Oysters, raw	100g/3½oz	190	270	51
53.	Scampi, fried	100g/3½oz	99	310	316
54.	Shrimp, canned	100g/3½oz	110	150	94
Meat					
55.	Bacon, gammon, grilled	100g/3½oz	9	260	228
56.	Beef, minced, stewed	100g/3½oz	18	170	229
57.	Beef sausage, grilled	100g/3½oz	73	210	265
58.	Beefburger, fried	100g/3½oz	33	250	264
59.	Lamb, leg, roast	100g/3½oz	8	200	266
60.	Pork chop, grilled	100g/3½oz	11	230	332
Poultry					
61.	Chicken, roast	100g/3½oz	9	210	148
62.	Duck, roast	100g/3½oz	13	200	189
63.	Goose, roast	100g/3½oz	10	270	319
64.	Turkey, roast	100g/3½oz	9	220	140
Cooked meat dishes					
65.	Beef steak pudding	100g/3½oz	110	140	223
66.	Moussaka	100g/3½oz	88	130	195
67.	Shepherd's pie	100g/3½oz	15	69	119
Soups					
68.	Chicken, cream of	100g/3½oz	27	27	58
69.	Mushroom, cream of	100g/3½oz	30	30	53
70.	Tomato, cream of	100g/3½oz	17	20	55

Item	Food	Amount	Ca (mg)	P (mg)	Calories
	FRUITS AND FRUIT PRODUCTS				
71.	Apples, eating	1 apple	4	8	46
72.	Apricots, canned	100g/3½oz	12	13	106
73.	Avocados (Fuerte)	1 avocado	30	62	446
74.	Bananas	1 banana	7	28	79
75.	Blackberries, raw	100g/3½oz	63	24	29
76.	Blackcurrants, stewed with sugar	100g/3½oz	47	34	59
77.	Cherries, eating, raw	100g/3½oz	16	17	47
78.	Damsons, stewed with sugar	100g/3½oz	17	13	69
79.	Dates, dried, without stones	12 dates	68	64	248
80.	Figs, dried	100g/3½oz	280	92	213
81.	Fruit salad, canned	100g/3½oz	8	10	95
82.	Gooseberries, stewed with sugar	100g/3½oz	22	27	50
83.	Grapes, black, raw	100g/3½oz	4	16	61
84.	Grapefruit, raw	½ fruit	17	16	22
85.	Greengages, raw	100g/3½oz	17	23	47
86.	Lemon juice, fresh	100g/3½oz	8	10	7
87.	Loganberries, raw	100g/3½oz	35	24	17
88.	Melon, canteloupe	½ melon	38	60	48
89.	watermelon	100g/3½oz	5	8	21
90.	Olives, in brine	25g/1oz	15	4	26
91.	Oranges	1 orange	41	24	35
92.	Orange juice, fresh	150ml/¼pt	18	33	57
93.	Peaches, raw	1 peach	5	19	37
94.	canned	100g/3½oz	4	10	87
95.	Pears, eating	1 pear	8	10	41
96.	Pineapple, canned	100g/3½oz	13	5	77
97.	Plums, raw	1 plum	7	11	25
98.	Prunes, stewed without sugar	100g/3½oz	19	42	82
99.	Raisins, dried	100g/3½oz	61	33	246
100.	Raspberries, raw	100g/3½oz	41	29	25
101.	Rhubarb, stewed with sugar	100g/3½oz	84	18	45

Item	Food	Amount	Ca (mg)	P (mg)	Calories
102.	Strawberries, raw	100g/3½oz	22	23	26

GRAINS AND GRAIN PRODUCTS

Item	Food	Amount	Ca (mg)	P (mg)	Calories
103.	Barley (pearl), raw	100g/3½oz	10	210	360
104.	Bran (wheat)	100g/3½oz	110	1200	206
105.	Cornflour	100g/3½oz	15	39	354
106.	Flour, wholemeal (100 per cent)	100g/3½oz	35	340	318
107.	brown (85 per cent) (fortified)	100g/3½oz	150	270	327
108.	white, plain (fortified)	100g/3½oz	150	110	350
109.	Macaroni, raw	100g/3½oz	26	150	370
110.	Oatmeal, raw	100g/3½oz	55	380	401
111.	Rice, polished, raw	100g/3½oz	4	100	361
112.	Spaghetti, raw	100g/3½oz	23	120	378
113.	canned in tomato sauce	100g/3½oz	21	30	59

Breads

Item	Food	Amount	Ca (mg)	P (mg)	Calories
114.	Wholemeal	100g/3½oz	23	230	216
115.	Brown	100g/3½oz	100	190	223
116.	White	100g/3½oz	100	97	233
117.	Malt	100g/3½oz	94	250	248
118.	Chapatis, without fat	100g/3½oz	60	120	202

Breakfast cereals

Item	Food	Amount	Ca (mg)	P (mg)	Calories
119.	All-Bran	100g/3½oz	74	900	273
120.	Cornflakes	100g/3½oz	3	47	368
121.	Muesli (commercial)	100g/3½oz	200	380	368
122.	Ready Brek	100g/3½oz	64	420	390
123.	Weetabix	100g/3½oz	33	300	340

Biscuits

Item	Food	Amount	Ca (mg)	P (mg)	Calories
124.	Chocolate	100g/3½oz	110	130	524
125.	Cream crackers	100g/3½oz	110	110	440
126.	Crispbread, rye	100g/3½oz	50	310	321
127.	Digestive, plain	100g/3½oz	110	130	471
128.	Ginger nuts	100g/3½oz	130	87	456

Item	Food	Amount	Ca (ma)	P (ma)	Calories
129.	Matzo	100g/3½oz	32	100	384
130.	Oatcakes	100g/3½oz	54	420	441
131.	Semi-sweet	100g/3½oz	120	84	457
132.	Shortbread	100g/3½oz	97	75	504
133.	Water biscuits	100g/3½oz	120	87	440

Cakes

Item	Food	Amount	Ca (ma)	P (ma)	Calories
134.	Fruit cake	100g/3½oz	60	110	354
135.	Gingerbread	100g/3½oz	210	91	373
136.	Madeira cake	100g/3½oz	42	120	393
137.	Swiss roll	100g/3½oz	44	220	302
138.	Victoria sponge	100g/3½oz	140	150	464

Buns and pastries

Item	Food	Amount	Ca (ma)	P (ma)	Calories
139.	Currant buns	100g/3½oz	90	65	302
140.	Jam tarts	100g/3½oz	62	47	384
141.	Pastry, shortcrust, cooked	100g/3½oz	110	79	527
142.	Scones	100g/3½oz	620	470	371

Puddings

Item	Food	Amount	Ca (ma)	P (ma)	Calories
143.	Bread and butter pudding	100g/3½oz	130	140	159
144.	Cheesecake	100g/3½oz	67	87	421
145.	Christmas pudding	100g/3½oz	87	93	304
146.	Custard tart	100g/3½oz	110	100	287
147.	Sponge pudding	100g/3½oz	210	190	344
148.	Treacle tart	100g/3½oz	65	51	371
149.	Yorkshire pudding	100g/3½oz	130	130	215

HERBS, SPICES AND SEEDS

Item	Food	Amount	Ca (ma)	P (ma)	Calories
150.	Allspice powder	5g/1tsp	33	n/a	13
151.	Anise seeds	5g/1tsp	32	n/a	17
152.	Caraway seeds	5g/1tsp	34	n/a	17
153.	Cardamom powder	5g/1tsp	19	n/a	16
154.	Chilli powder	5g/1tsp	14	n/a	16
155.	Cinnamon powder	5g/1tsp	61	n/a	13
156.	Coriander leaves, dried	5g/1tsp	62	n/a	14
157.	seeds	5g/1tsp	35	n/a	15

Item	Food	Amount	Ca (mg)	P (mg)	Calories
158.	Cumin seeds	5g/1 tsp	47	n/a	19
159.	Curry powder	5g/1 tsp	24	n/a	16
160.	Dill seeds	5g/1 tsp	76	n/a	15
161.	Fennel seeds	5g/1 tsp	60	n/a	17
162.	Fenugreek seeds	5g/1 tsp	9	n/a	16
163.	Ginger powder	5g/1 tsp	5	7	13
164.	Mustard powder	5g/1 tsp	16	9	23
165.	seeds	5g/1 tsp	26	n/a	23
166.	Nutmeg powder	5g/1 tsp	9	n/a	26
167.	Oregano powder	5g/1 tsp	79	n/a	15
168.	Paprika	5g/1 tsp	9	n/a	14
169.	Parsley, dried	5g/1 tsp	73	n/a	14
170.	Rosemary, dried	5g/1 tsp	64	n/a	17
171.	Saffron/kaisar	5g/1 tsp	6	n/a	15
172.	Sesame seeds	5g/1 tsp	7	n/a	29
173.	Turmeric powder	5g/1 tsp	9	n/a	18

LEGUMES AND RELATED PRODUCTS

Item	Food	Amount	Ca (mg)	P (mg)	Calories
174.	Beans, baked, canned in tomato sauce	100g/3½oz	45	91	64
175.	broad, boiled	100g/3½oz	21	99	48
176.	butter, boiled	100g/3½oz	19	87	95
177.	French, boiled	100g/3½oz	39	15	7
178.	haricot, boiled	100g/3½oz	65	120	93
179.	mung, cooked (dahl)	100g/3½oz	34	100	106
180.	red kidney, boiled	100g/3½oz	140	410	272
181.	runner, boiled	100g/3½oz	22	41	19
182.	Lentils, split, boiled	100g/3½oz	13	77	99
183.	Peanuts, fresh	100g/3½oz	61	370	570
184.	Peanut butter	100g/3½oz	37	330	623
185.	Peas, fresh, raw	100g/3½oz	15	100	67
186.	frozen, boiled	100g/3½oz	31	84	41
187.	Soya flour	100g/3½oz	210	600	447
188.	Soya milk (unfortified)	100g/3½oz	5	n/a	39
189.	Tofu (beancurd)	100g/3½oz	507	n/a	70

Item	Food	Amount	Ca (mg)	P (mg)	Calories
NUTS					
190.	Almonds	100g/3½oz	250	440	565
191.	Brazils	100g/3½oz	180	590	619
192.	Chestnuts	100g/3½oz	46	74	170
193.	Cobs or hazels	100g/3½oz	44	230	380
194.	Coconut, fresh	100g/3½oz	13	94	351
	Peanuts. See Legumes.				
195.	Walnuts	100g/3½oz	61	510	525
OILS AND FATS					
196.	Butter	100g/3½oz	15	24	740
197.	Cod-liver oil	100g/3½oz	tr.	tr.	899
198.	Dripping (beef)	100g/3½oz	1	13	891
199.	Lard	100g/3½oz	1	3	891
200.	Lowfat spread	100g/3½oz	tr.	tr.	366
201.	Margarine	100g/3½oz	4	12	730
202.	Olive oil	100g/3½oz	tr.	tr.	900
203.	Suet, shredded	100g/3½oz	tr.	tr.	826
204.	Vegetable oils	100g/3½oz	tr.	tr.	899
SAUCES, DRESSINGS AND CONDIMENTS					
205.	Bread sauce	50g/2oz	60	50	55
206.	Brown sauce, bottled	25g/1oz	11	9	25
207.	Cheese sauce	50g/2oz	130	95	99
208.	French dressing	25g/1oz	1	2	164
209.	Mayonnaise	25g/1oz	4	15	179
210.	Pepper	5g/1tsp	6	6	15
211.	Salad cream	25g/1oz	8	22	78
212.	Salt, table	5g/1tsp	1	tr.	0
213.	White sauce, savoury	50g/2oz	70	55	75
SUGARS, PRESERVES AND SWEETS					
Sugars					
214.	Molasses, blackstrap	25g/1oz	171	21	53
215.	Sugar, demerara	25g/1oz	13	5	98
216.	white	25g/1oz	tr.	tr.	98
217.	Syrup, golden	25g/1oz	6	5	74

Item	Food	Amount	Ca (mg)	P (mg)	Calories
218.	Treacle, black	25g/1oz	125	8	64

Preserves

Item	Food	Amount	Ca (mg)	P (mg)	Calories
219.	Honey	25g/1oz	1	4	72
220.	Jam, with seeds	25g/1oz	6	4	65
221.	Lemon curd, home-made	25g/1oz	4	15	72
222.	Marmalade	25g/1oz	9	3	65
223.	Mincemeat	25g/1oz	7	4	59

Sweets

Item	Food	Amount	Ca (mg)	P (mg)	Calories
224.	Boiled sweets	25g/1oz	1	3	82
225.	Chocolate, milk	25g/1oz	55	60	132
226.	plain	25g/1oz	9	35	131
227.	Fruit gums	25g/1oz	90	1	43
228.	Liquorice allsorts	25g/1oz	16	7	78
229.	Peppermints	25g/1oz	2	tr.	98
230.	Toffees, mixed	25g/1oz	24	16	107

VEGETABLES AND VEGETABLE PRODUCTS

Item	Food	Amount	Ca (mg)	P (mg)	Calories
231.	Artichokes, globe	100g/3½oz	19	17	7
232.	Jerusalem	100g/3½oz	30	33	18
233.	Asparagus, boiled	100g/3½oz	13	42	9
234.	Aubergine, raw	100g/3½oz	10	12	14
	Beans. See Legumes.				
235.	Beetroot, boiled	100g/3½oz	30	36	44
236.	Broccoli, boiled	100g/3½oz	76	60	18
237.	Brussels sprouts, boiled	100g/3½oz	25	51	18
238.	Cabbage, red	100g/3½oz	53	32	20
239.	Savoy, boiled	100g/3½oz	53	27	9
240.	spring, boiled	100g/3½oz	30	32	7
241.	white, raw	100g/3½oz	44	36	22
242.	Carrots, old, boiled	100g/3½oz	37	17	19
243.	Cauliflower, boiled	100g/3½oz	18	32	9
244.	Celery, raw	100g/3½oz	52	32	8
245.	Chicory, raw	100g/3½oz	18	21	9
246.	Cucumber, raw	100g/3½oz	23	24	10
247.	Garlic, raw	25g/1oz	4	n/a	29
248.	Horseradish, raw	25g/1oz	30	17	15

Item	Food	Amount	Ca (mg)	P (mg)	Calories
249.	Leeks, boiled	100g/3½oz	61	28	24
250.	Lettuce, raw	100g/3½oz	23	27	12
251.	Marrow, boiled	100g/3½oz	14	13	7
252.	Mushrooms, raw	100g/3½oz	3	140	13
253.	Mustard and cress, raw	50g/2oz	33	33	5
254.	Okra, raw	100g/3½oz	70	60	17
255.	Onions, raw	100g/3½oz	31	30	23
256.	boiled	100g/3½oz	24	16	13
257.	fried	100g/3½oz	61	59	345
258.	spring, raw	50g/2oz	70	12	17
259.	Parsley, raw	25g/1oz	82	32	5
260.	Parsnips, boiled	100g/3½oz	36	32	56
	Peas. See Legumes.				
261.	Peppers, green, raw	50g/2oz	4	12	7
262.	Potatoes, old, mashed	100g/3½oz	12	32	119
263.	baked	100g/3½oz	8	39	85
264.	chips	100g/3½oz	14	72	253
265.	Potato instant powder, as served	100g/3½oz	20	48	70
266.	Potato crisps	50g/2oz	18	65	266
267.	Radishes, raw	50g/2oz	22	13	7
268.	Salsify, boiled	100g/3½oz	60	53	18
269.	Seakale, boiled	100g/3½oz	48	34	8
270.	Spinach, boiled	100g/3½oz	600	93	30
271.	Spring greens, boiled	100g/3½oz	86	31	10
272.	Swedes, boiled	100g/3½oz	42	18	18
273.	Sweetcorn, boiled	100g/3½oz	4	120	123
274.	canned	100g/3½oz	3	67	76
275.	Sweet potatoes, boiled	100g/3½oz	21	44	85
276.	Tomatoes, raw	100g/3½oz	13	21	14
277.	canned	100g/3½oz	9	22	12
278.	Turnips, boiled	100g/3½oz	55	19	14
279.	Turnip tops, boiled	100g/3½oz	98	45	11
280.	Watercress, raw	50g/2oz	110	26	7
281.	Yams, boiled	100g/3½oz	9	33	119

Item	Food	Amount	Ca (mg)	P (mg)	Calories
MISCELLANEOUS FOODS					
282.	Baking powder	5g/1 tsp	565*	421*	8
283.	Marmite	5g/1 tsp	5	85	9
284.	Vinegar	15ml/1 tbsp	2	5	1
285.	Yeast, baker's, compressed	50g/2 oz	12	195	26
BEVERAGES					
Alcoholic					
286.	Beer, brown ale, bottled	300ml/½ pt	21	33	84
287.	draught bitter	300ml/½ pt	33	39	96
288.	strong ale	300ml/½ pt	42	120	216
289.	Cider, dry	300ml/½ pt	24	9	108
290.	Spirits	50ml/2 fl oz	tr.	tr.	111
291.	Wine, red	100ml/4 fl oz	7	14	68
292.	white, dry	100ml/4 fl oz	9	6	66
Non-alcoholic					
293.	Bovril	5g/1 tsp	2	29	9
294.	Chocolate, drinking	150ml/¼ pt	49	285	549
295.	Coca-Cola	150ml/¼ pt	6	22	58
296.	Coffee, infusion	150ml/¼ pt	3	3	3
297.	Lemonade, bottled	150ml/¼ pt	7	tr.	31
298.	Milk, cow's, whole	150ml/¼ pt	180	142	98
299.	skimmed	150ml/¼ pt	195	150	50
	For other milks, see *Dairy Products*.				
300.	Orange juice, canned, unsweetened	150ml/¼ pt	13	22	49
301.	Tea, Indian, infusion	150ml/¼ pt	tr.	1	1
302.	Tomato juice, canned	150ml/¼ pt	15	30	24

*variable, depending on brand.

REFERENCES

Albanese, Anthony A. *et al.*, *Calcium throughout the Lifecycle* (National Dairy Council, 1978)

Asimov, Isaac, *The Human Body* (Houghton, 1963)

Bauer, Cathy and Andersen, Juel, *The Tofu Cookbook* (Rodale Press, 1979)

Cann, C. E. *et al.*, 'Spinal Mineral Loss in Oopherectomized Women' in *Journal of the American Medical Association*, Vol. 244, 1980

Cooke, Cynthia W. and Dworkin, Susan, *The Ms. Guide to a Woman's Health* (Doubleday, Garden City, New York, 1979)

Cutler, Winnifred Berg *et al.*, *Menopause, A Guide for Women and the Men Who Love Them* (Norton, New York, 1983)

Daniell, H. W., 'Osteoporosis of the Slender Smoker' in *Archives of Internal Medicine*, Vol. 136, 1976

Davis, Adelle, *Let's Stay Healthy*, edited 1981 by Ann Gildroy (Harcourt, Brace, Jovanovich, New York, 1981)

Department of Health and Social Security, *Eating for Health* (H.M.S.O., 1978)

De Vries, Herbert A. with Hales, Dianne, *Fitness after 50* (Scribner, New York, 1982)

FAO/WHO Expert Group, Technical Report Series No. 230, *Calcium Requirements*, (1962)

FAO/WHO Ad Hoc Expert Committee, *Protein Intake* (1973)

Frisch, R. E. *et al.*, 'Delayed Menarche and Amenorrhea of College Athletes in relation to onset of training' in *Journal of the American Medical Association*, Vol. 246, 1981

Gould, Roy, *Going Sour, The Science and Politics of Acid Rain* (Birkhäuser, Boston, 1985)

Heaney, Robert P. *et al.*, 'Calcium Balance and Calcium Requirements in Middle-Aged Women' in *The American Journal of Clinical Nutrition*, Vol. 30, 1977

Heaney, Robert P. *et al.*, 'Menopausal Changes in Bone Remodelling' in *The Journal of Laboratory and Clinical Medicine*, Vol. 92, 1978

Heaney, Robert P. *et al.*, 'Menopausal Changes in Calcium Balance Performance' in *The Journal of Laboratory and Clinical Medicine*, Vol. 92, 1978

Helferich, William and Westhoff, Dennis, *All About Yogurt* (Prentice-Hall, Englewood Cliffs, New Jersey, 1980)

James, W. *et al.*, 'Calcium Binding by Dietary Fibre' in *The Lancet*, Vol. 638, 1978

Leonard, Jon N. *et al.*, *Live Longer Now, The First 100 Years of Your Life* (Grosset and Dunlap, 1974)

Marcus, Robert, 'The Relationship of Dietary Calcium to the Maintenance of Skeletal Integrity in Man – an Interface of Endocrinology and Nutrition' in *Metabolism*, Vol. 31, No. 1, 1982

Marcus, Robert *et al.*, 'Menstrual Function and Bone Mass in Elite Women Distance Runners' in *Annals of Internal Medicine*, Vol. 102, No. 2, 1985

Matkovic, V. *et al.*, 'Bone Status and Fracture Rates in Two Regions of Yugoslavia' in *The American Journal of Clinical Nutrition*, Vol. 32, 1979

Mayer, Jean, *A Diet for Living* (D. McKay Co., 1975)

McConkey, B. *et al.*, 'Transparent Skin and Osteoporosis. A Study in Patients with Rheumatoid Disease' in *Annals of Rheumatic Diseases*, Vol. 24, 1965

McQueen-Williams, Morvyth and Apisson, Barbara, *A Diet for 100 Healthy Happy Years* (Prentice-Hall, Englewood Cliffs, New Jersey, 1977)

Ministry of Agriculture, Fisheries and Food. McCance and Widdowson's *The Composition of Foods*, 4th edition by A. A. Paul and D. A. T. Southgate of the Medical Research Council (H.M.S.O., 1978)

Ministry of Agriculture, Fisheries and Food. Second Supplement, *Immigrant Foods* by S. P. Tan *et al* (H.M.S.O., 1985)

Ministry of Agriculture, Fisheries and Food, *Manual of Nutrition* (H.M.S.O., 1976)

Ministry of Agriculture, Fisheries and Food, *Survey of Cadmium in Food* (H.M.S.O., 1983)

NASA, *A Brief Review of Space Flight Calcium Metabolism* (General Electric, 1978)

National Academy of Sciences, *Recommended Dietary Allowances* (1980)

National Institutes of Health, Statement of Consensus Development Conference on Osteoporosis (1984)

Notelovitz, Morris and Ware, Marsha, *Stand Tall! The Informed Woman's*

Guide to Preventing Osteoporosis (Triad Publishing Co., Gainesville, Florida, 1982)

Pennington, Jean A. T. and Church, Helen Nichols, *Food Values of Portions Commonly Used*, 13th revised edition (J. B. Lippincott Co., Philadelphia, 1980)

Recker, Robert R. *et al.*, 'Effect of Estrogens and Calcium Carbonate on Bone Loss in Postmenopausal Women' in *Annals of Internal Medicine*, Vol. 87, No. 6, 1977

Stott, Susan, and Gray, D. H., 'The Incidence of Femoral Neck Fractures in New Zealand' in *New Zealand Medical Journal*, No. 651, 1980

Van Amerongen, C., *Book of the Body: The Way Things Work* (Simon and Schuster, 1979)

United States Department of Agriculture, *Nutritive Value of Foods* (Revised 1981)

United States Department of Agriculture, *Nutritive Value of American Foods in Common Units* (1975)

Index